Ninety - Nine Nifty Notes

from the

Nine Lives Experts:

A Primer for Revivors

Chris Collins
Marian Brickner Collaborator

Revivor LLC
301 Sovereign Court, Suite 200
Ballwin, MO 63011
www.revivor.net

Cover and book design by Chris Collins.
Typeset in Neometric.

Ninety - Nine Nifty Notes from the Nine Lives
Experts: A Primer for Revivors.

Summary: Notes gives options for looking at life
differently using relaxation, meditation, calm, humor
and courage to heal when faced with a terminal or
frightening diagnosis.

Fiction, self-reliance, options on intuitive healing

Dedication:

This book is dedicated
to all Revivors around the
world who heal despite
being told it's impossible.

Table of CONTEXT

Self Knowledge:
1, 20, 37, 38, 45, 48, 49, 51, 54, 55, 60,77, 78, 79, 83, 84, 88 ,95

Accept the Unknowable:
2, 20, 40, 44, 46, 56, 79, 80, 81, 84, 85

Slow down, nap:
3, 19, 22, 28, 32, 42, 50, 59, 67, 71

Exercize:
4, 33, 41, 98

Table of CONTEXT
(Cont'd)

Focus:
5, 17, 18, 25, 27, 65, 66, 69,
71, 86, 91, 92, 93, 95, 99

Eat and Drink Well:
6, 7, 8, 30, 47

Meditate:
9, 52, 67

Play:
10, 11, 12, 14, 23, 43, 63, 73, 98

Appreciate:
13, 36, 39, 89

Table of CONTEXT
(Cont'd)

Pain:

15, 26

Trust:

16, 21, 29, 31, 34, 35, 37, 57, 62, 64
68, 72, 74, 75, 76, 79, 80, 81, 82, 88,
87, 92, 94, 97

Love:

24, 53, 58, 61, 70, 77, 87, 90, 96

Acknowledgments

A very furry thank you to Joseph Z. Starr who helped to give a good tempo and correct wording to these notes. I purr in your general direction, Joe!

Thanks also goes to Marian Brickner for the hours, days and weeks it took and the patience she had when there was nothing going on.
She was also my cat translator.

Thanks to Badria Jazairi who has shown me how cats really feel when they are totally loved like her cats are. Your cats are exquisite and so are you Badria.

Acknowledgments (cont'd)

Thanks go to all the photographers who produced these pictures through www.pixabay.com. In each image you will find a number at the bottom, and if you go into pixabay, you will easily find the image and the photographer should you want to pursue more of them. When people give freely of their talents, and their love, this is what can happen.

Ultimate gratitude goes to the Universe who put these words into my head (over 48 hours) and suggested I use feline wisdom

Acknowledgments (cont'd)

to put across these concepts.

These notes are for those of us
who are working towards and playing
with the idea of staying alive when
the odds are majorly stacked
against us.

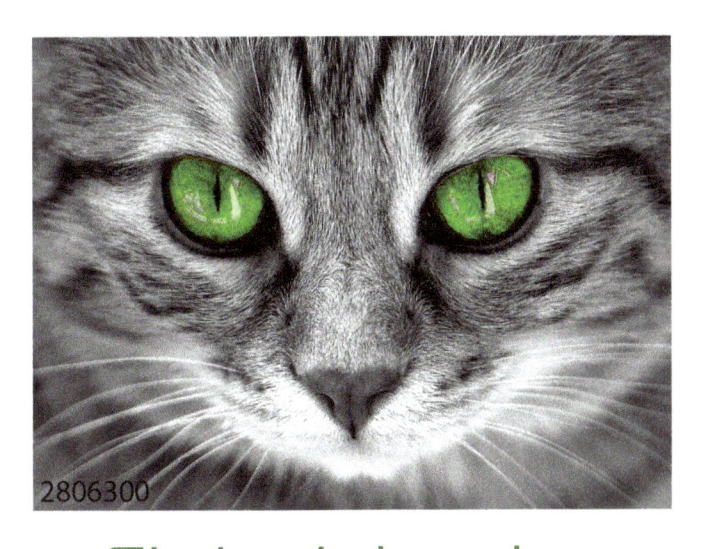

2806300

Study what you love
and why. There is no
harder job on the planet
than to completely
know
and accept
ourselves.
- Hans

It is neither possible nor desirable to understand everything all the time. Get comfortable being in the dark and continue on.

- Raven

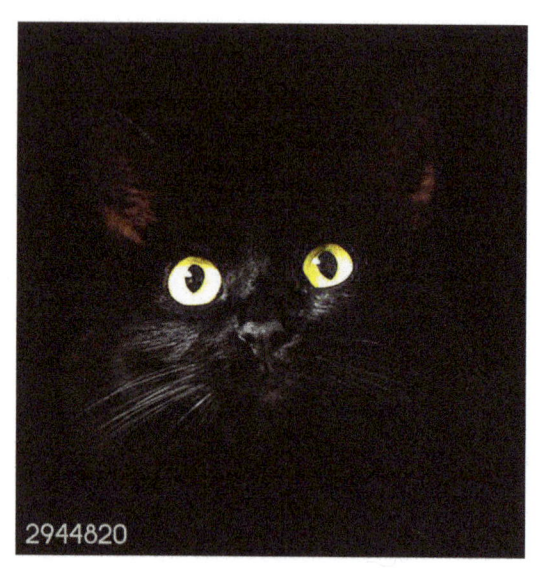

2944820

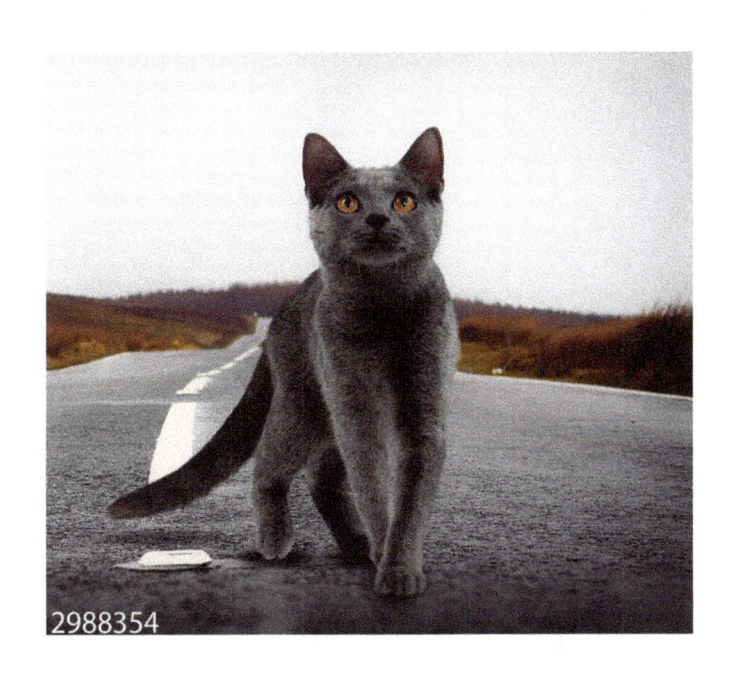

2988354

Sniff, watch, take one
slow step.
For the long haul,
it invariably pays off.

- Desdemona

Devise ways to exercize,
both body and soul.
If you can't move much on the
outside, figure out how to move
on the inside.
You can do this!

- Remington

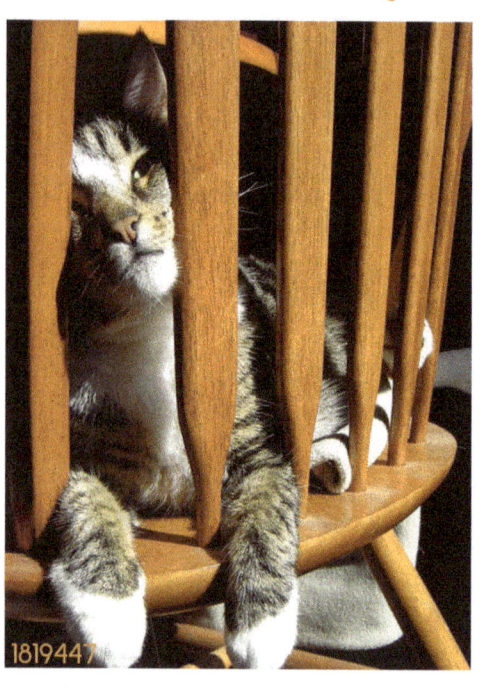

- 4 -

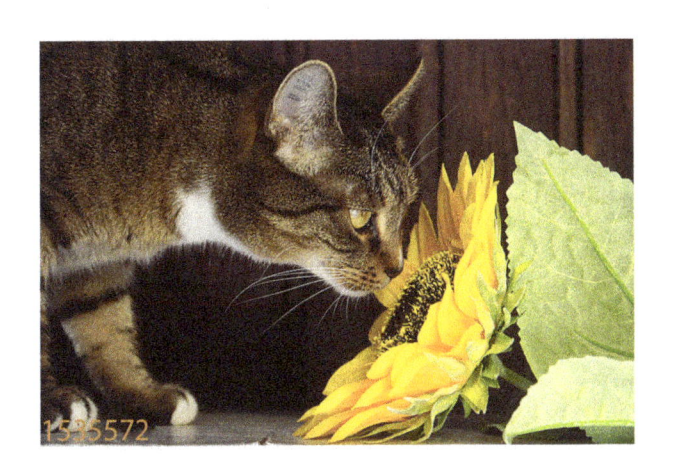

Focus on each joyful
moment as it comes
about. Don't worry.
It takes a while
to master this.
Practice, practice.

- Philamena

Eat only things that
a) taste exceptionally
interesting
or b) are the best for
your lovely body.
Just because everyone else
eats just any old thing
doesn't mean you have to.

- Charlie

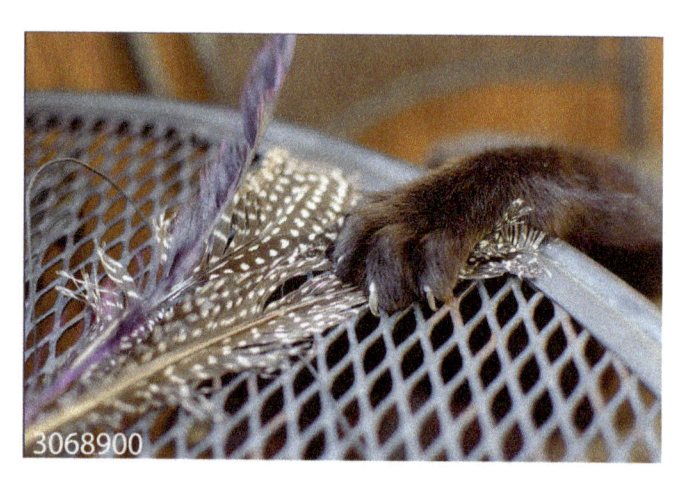

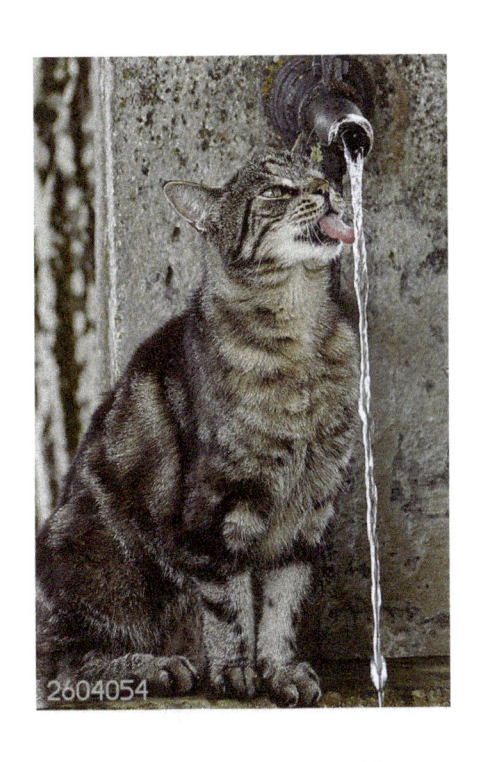

Drink water often.
From where it flows
does not matter, as long
as it's reasonably clean.

- Guinness

Do nothing else while
eating but bury your face
in your food and chew
every morsel well.
Tall sided bowls help to
reverberate the sound.

- Hilda

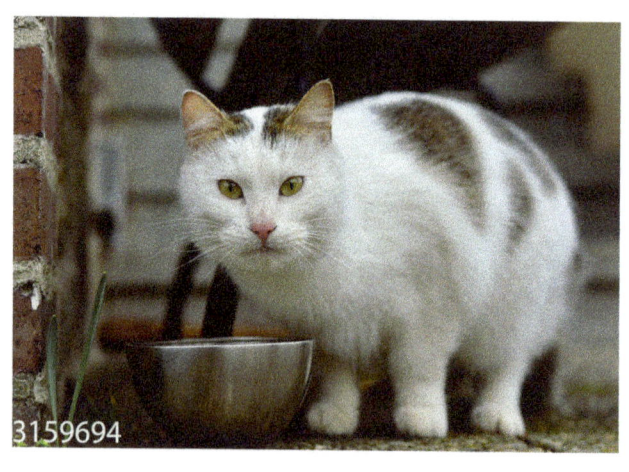

3159694

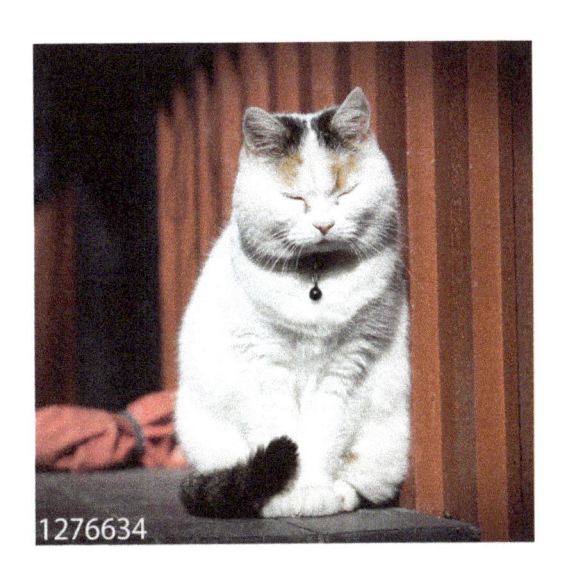

1276634

Sit in the sunlight,
for study and meditation,
while breathing
well and deep.
This is hard to stop.
Pace yourself.

- Opus

Play with pretty and
fun things, which might
include people,
as often as possible.

- Claudette

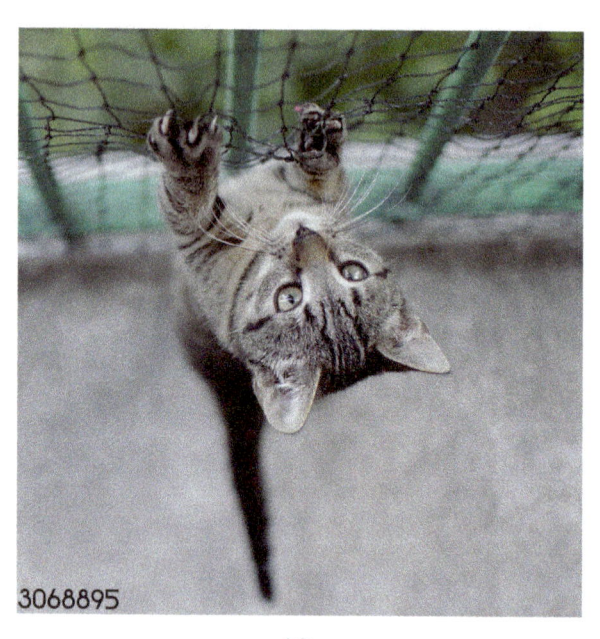

3068895

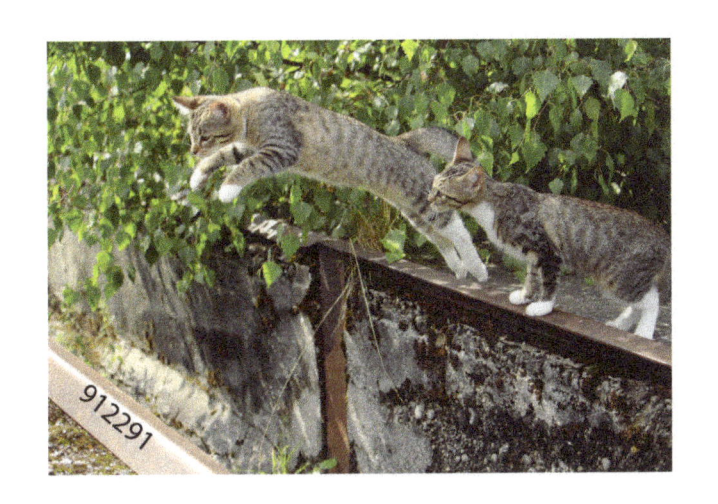

Play every day.
For at least
a little while.

- Heidi and Heloise

Play in feathers.
Play in greenery,
play in cat wheels.
Quit before
someone
gets dizzy.

- Muriel

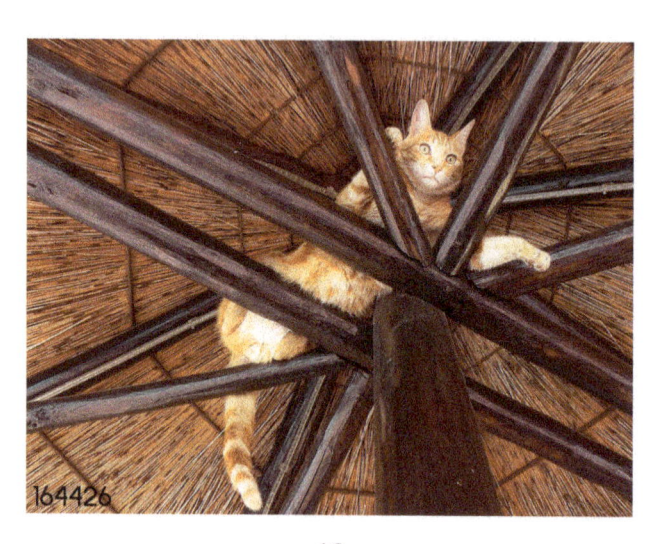

164426

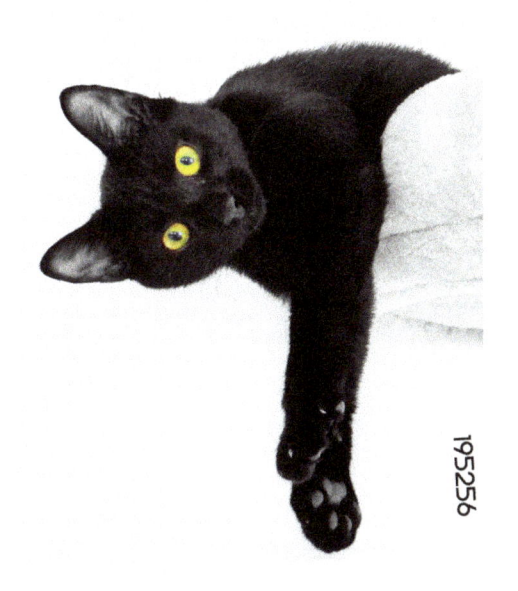

195256

Show appreciation
and gratitude for this
mesmerizing day,
by purring or not.

- Raven

Ever so slightly,
tap a friend on the nose
for no reason.
It will make you happy
and encourage
them to wonder.

- Remington

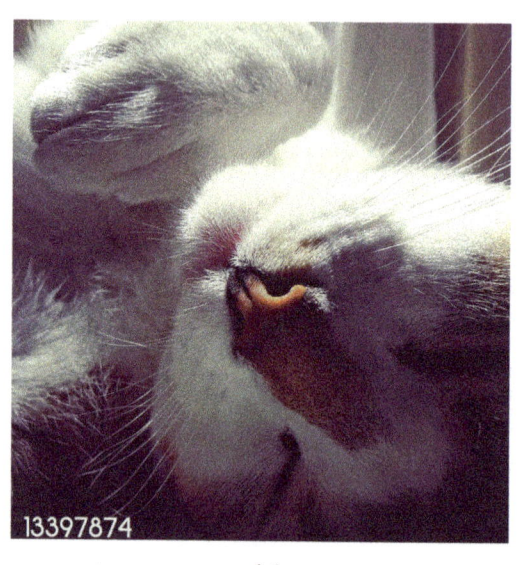

13397874

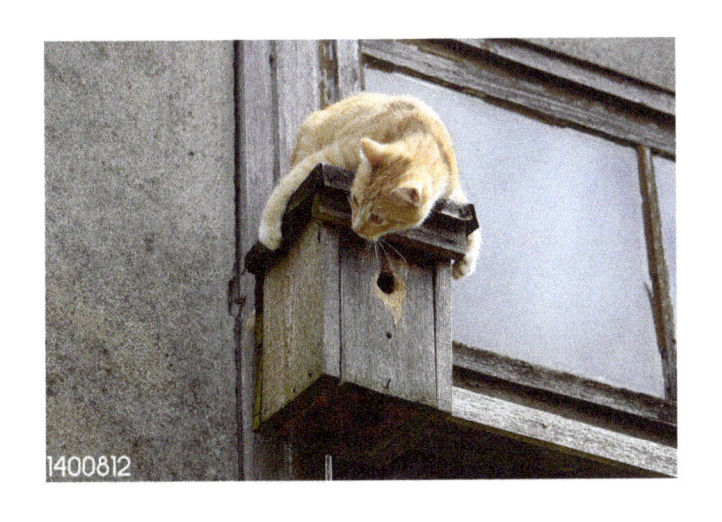

Pain allows perspective,
but only in hindsight.
Go ahead
and jump.

- Socrates

Don't be influenced
by what others
are supposedly thinking.
Go about
your business.

- Millicent

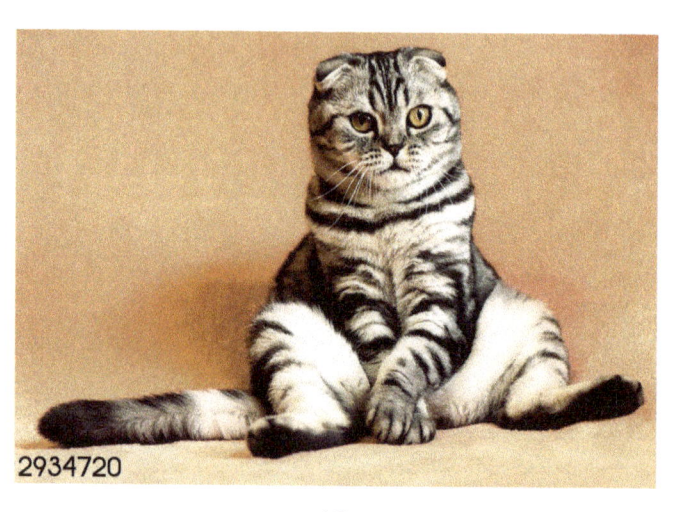

2934720

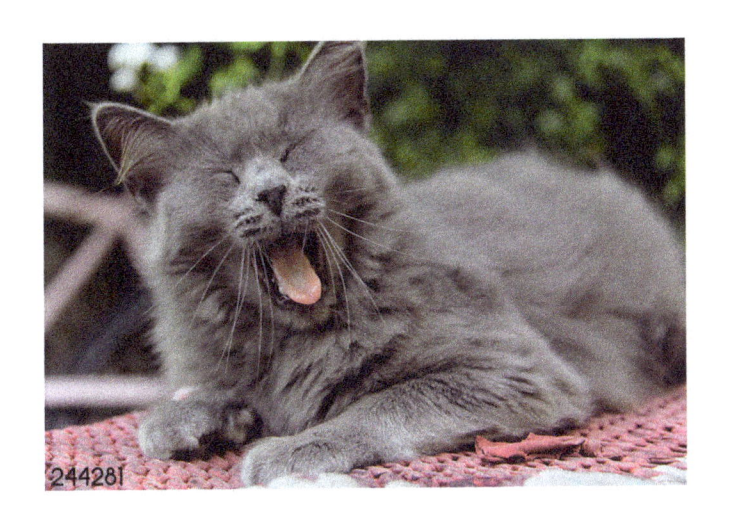

Ignore dire prophesies
about you,
or about others.
Go about
your business.

- Armani

When faced with the
eternal question,
"Am I living or am I dying?",
look out the window at Life.
You couldn't do that if
you weren't still here.
Go about your business.

- Sophie

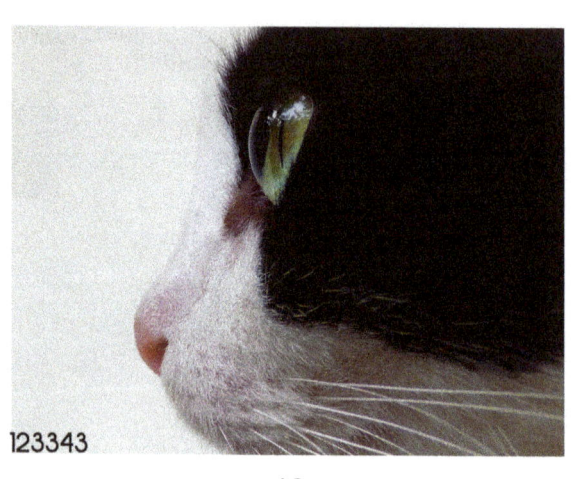

123343

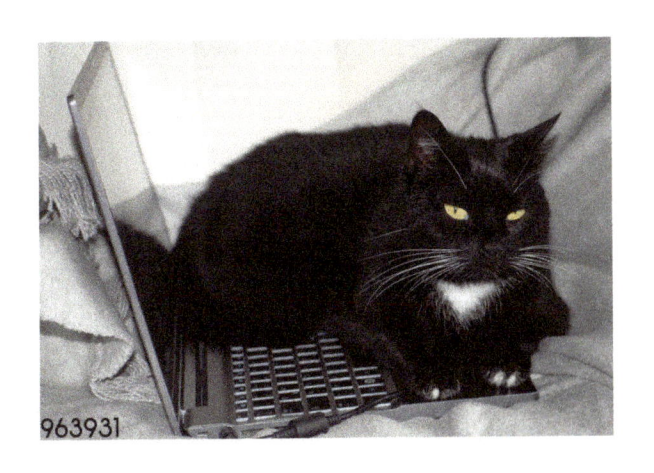

963931

Computers can be a great
tool for finding information,
but don't get addicted
to the screen.
You may, of course, get
addicted to the keyboard.
It's a perfect place
for a nap.
                        -Tasha

Assume that healing has
already begun.
Allow yourself to think
this continuously.
No one knows why we
heal, we just do.

- Purrscilla

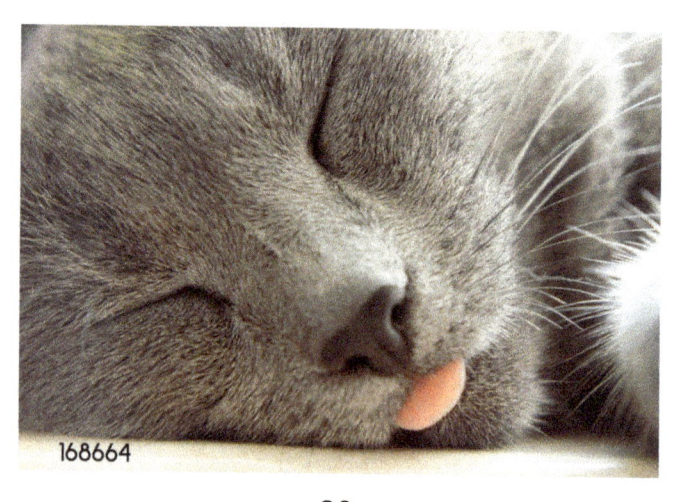

168664

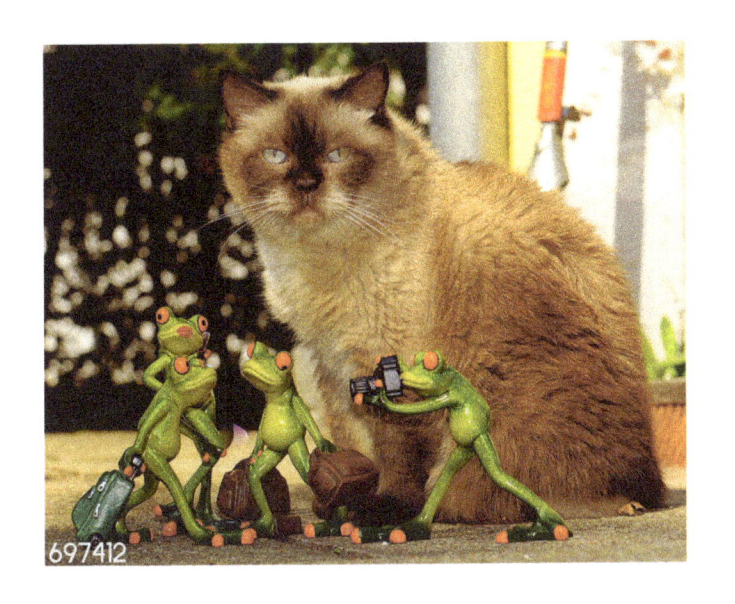

Stand guard for
others by being,
not by doing.

- Riley

Sleep in someone
else's bed.
It usually has a nice
curve to it.

- Willow

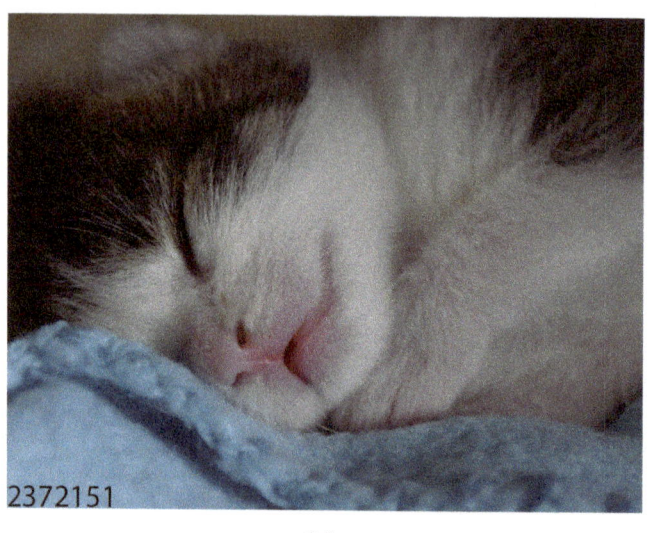

2372151

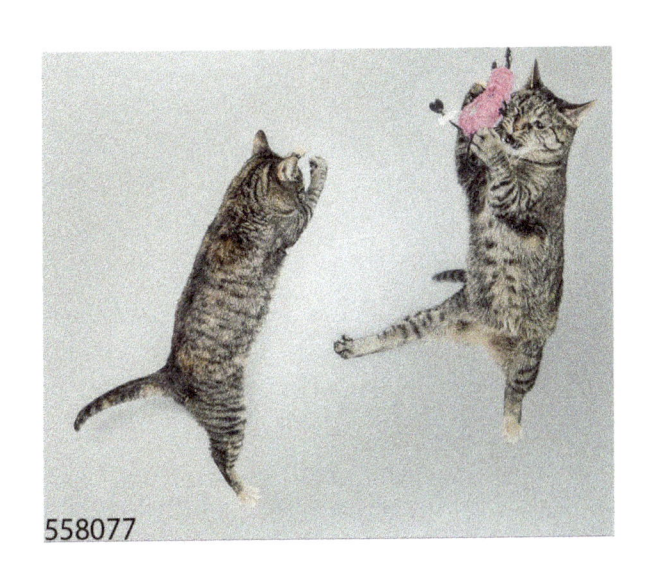

558077

Play with others
who are also healing.
They understand
how to have fun
even when
owies are present.

- Bruce and Bruno

Love others without them knowing,
sometimes from afar.
You will feel wonderful
all the time.
They might not know it the outside,
but on the inside,
it will manifest feats
of excellence
and perfect timing.

- Angelica

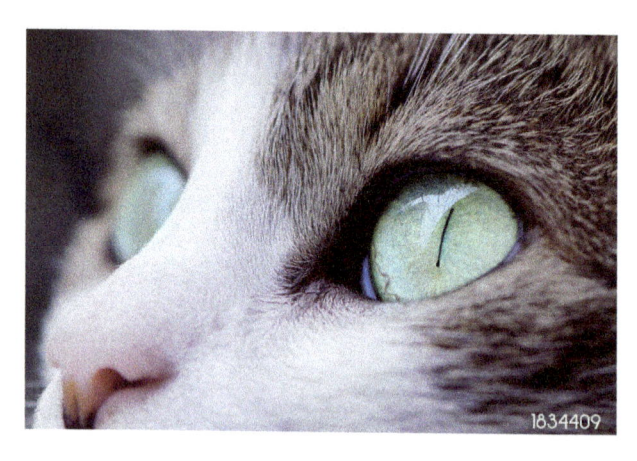

1834409

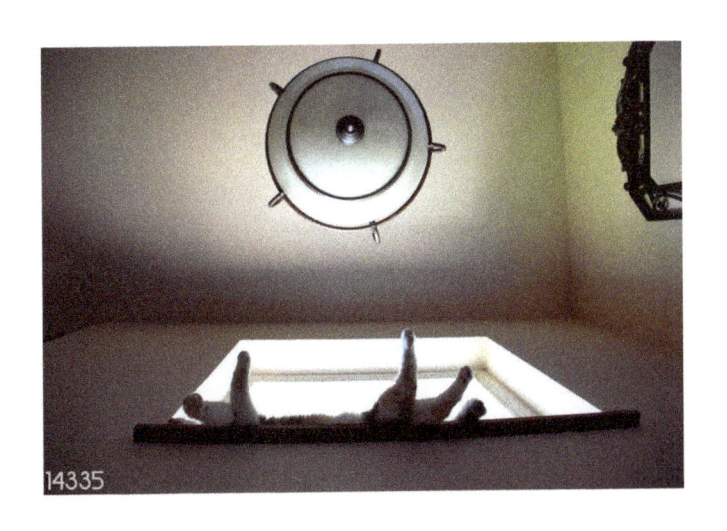

14335

Analyze the facts or use instincts
before making a healing
decision. CEERR.
Center oneself, experiment,
experience, results?
Repeat.
Of course, we always
land on our feet.

- Catalina

Trying hard at anything is not fun and there is no need. But if you still want to, go ahead. Doing things the hard way is the easy way to procrastinate.

- Victoria

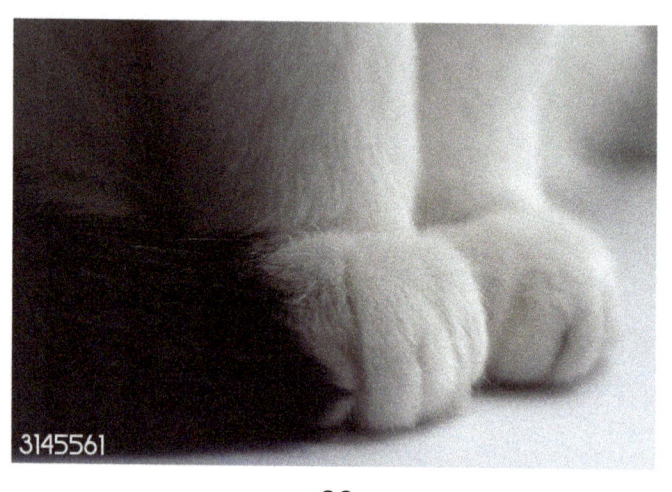

3145561

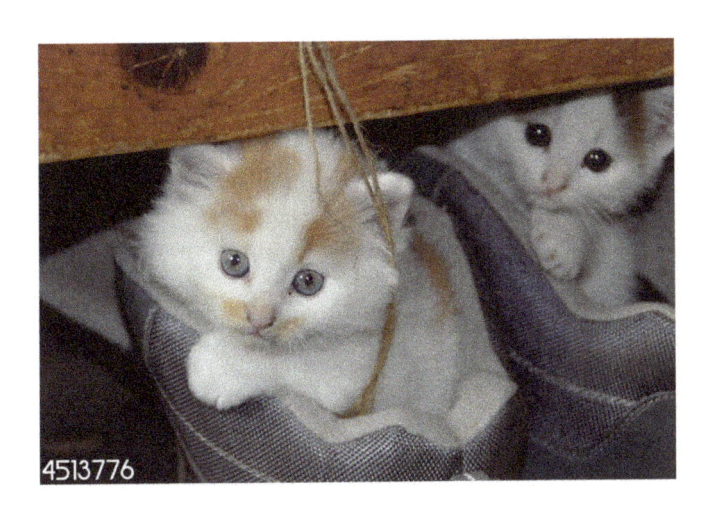

Search out only what
is truly helpful.
Celebrate each step to healing.
Discard, in a kind manner, the rest
or pitch like so much litter.

- Annabelle and Annaliese

Sample your options to
determine their worth.
You will know
when you have
sampled enough.

- Scruffia

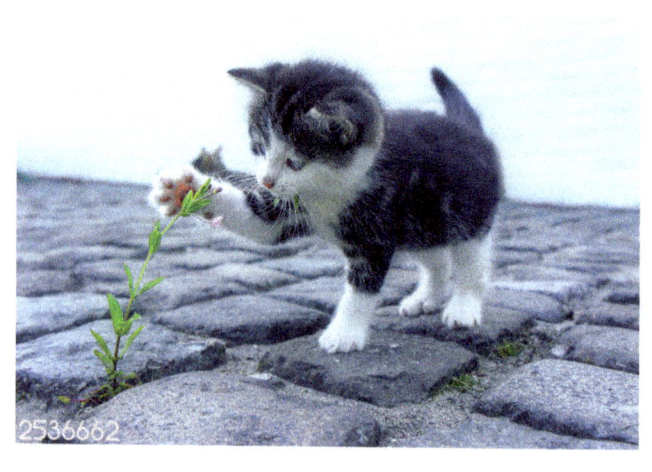

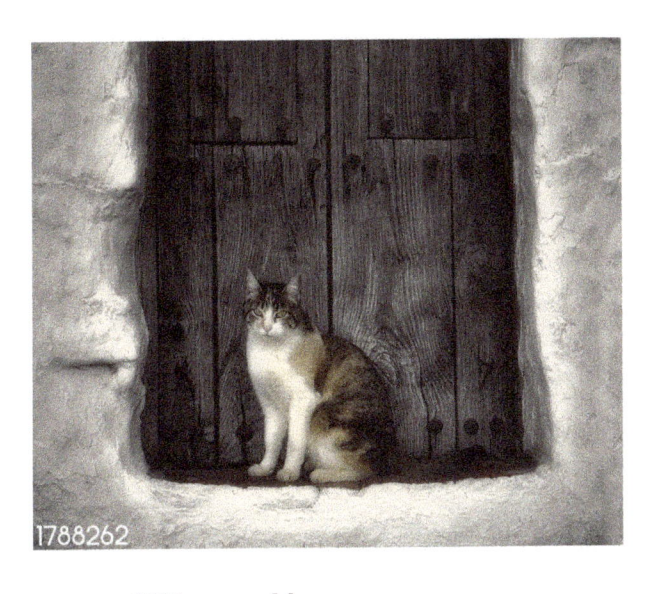

Stay the course.
You will find your way.
When the course changes,
your door,
the one just for you,
will open.

- Myrtle

Eating greens
is not always
enjoyable.
But it is
a daily necessity.

- Nigel -

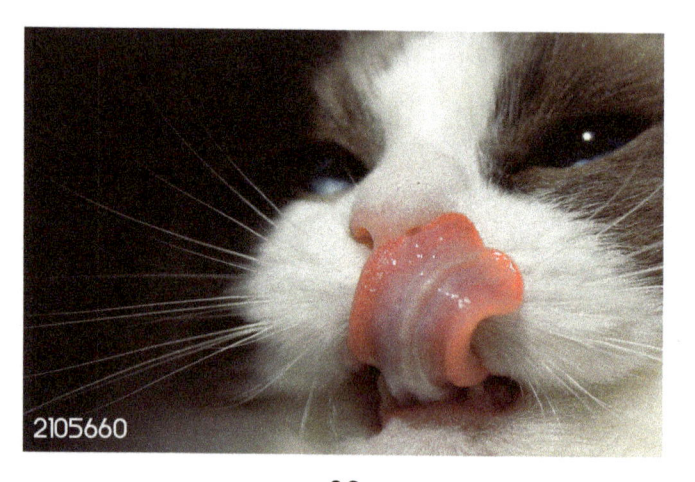

2105660

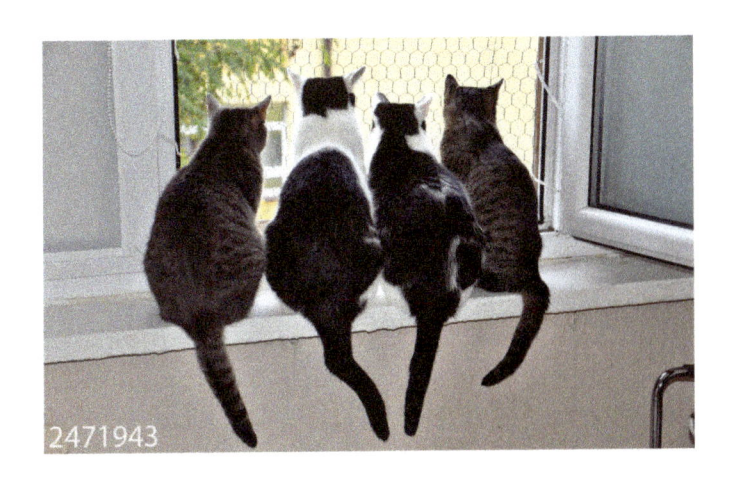

If you unintentionally
misstep upon another,
they will let you know,
not to worry.

- The Trance Family

Wait. It is always a good time to wait when we are called upon to do so. Lots can be done while we wait. Not to worry.

- Wampuss -

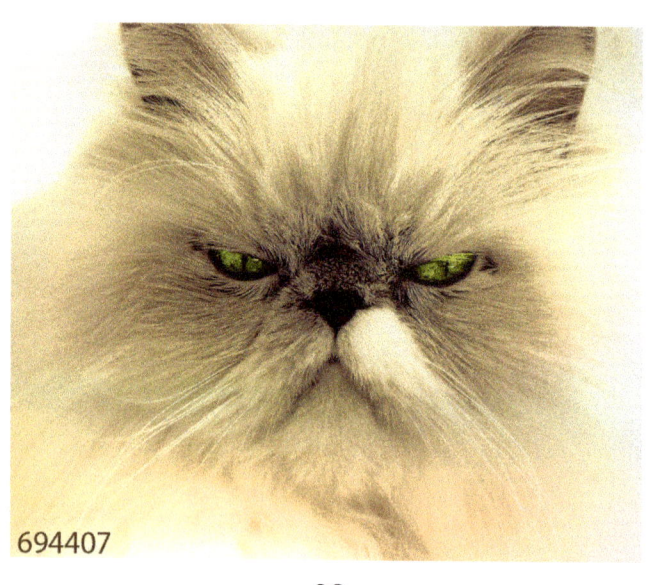

694407

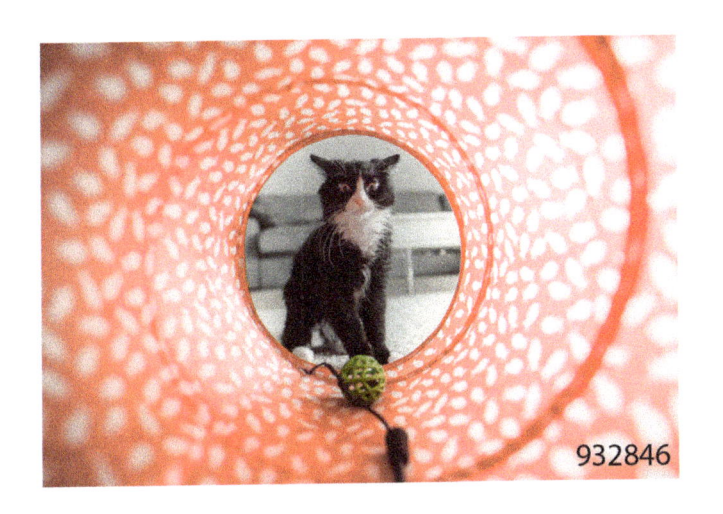

932846

Keep stepping forward,
sometimes backward.
Your steps work fine
either way.
Not to worry.

- Phineas

Things are not often what
they seem.
Pain doesn't always
connote a problem.
Often it is a
healing pain.

- Kali

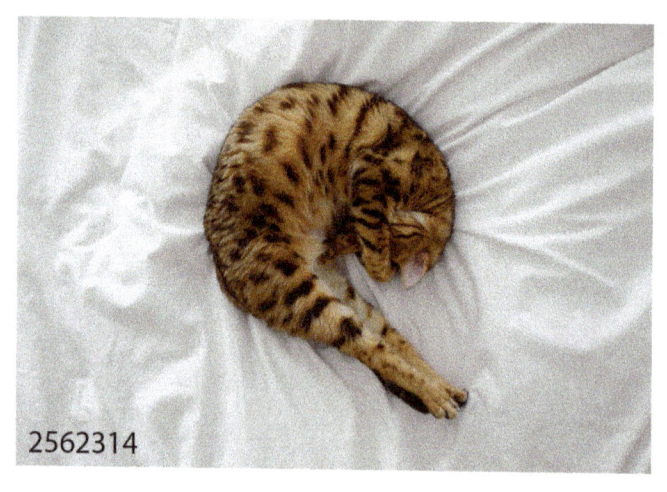

2562314

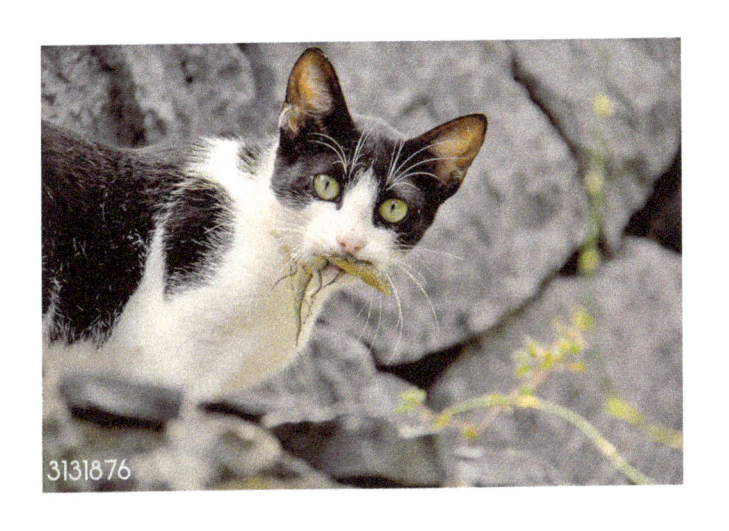

3131876

Don't expect too much
appreciation from others
when bringing them gifts.
They are busier
than you think.

- Herkimer

Whatever is at your disposal at this moment is plenty. Look around. Be amazed. Look again.

- The Pandora Kits

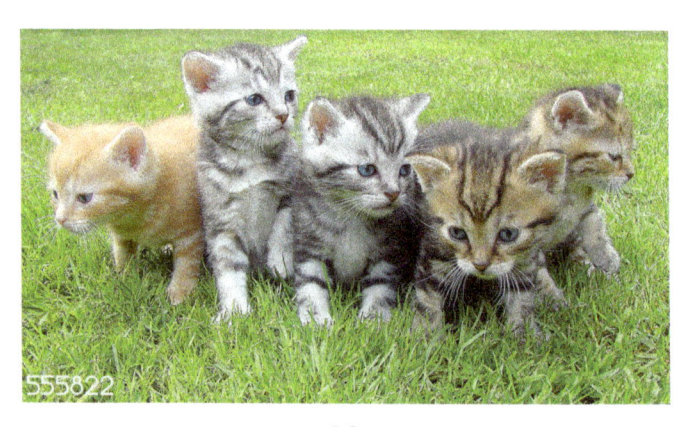

555822

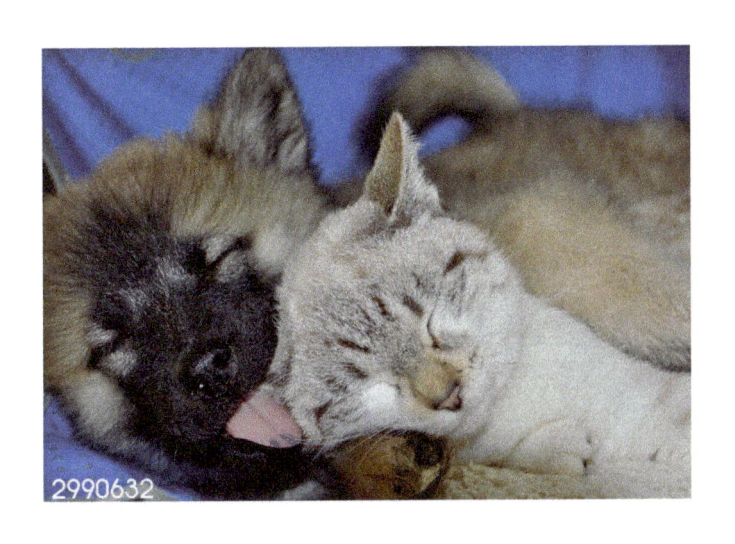

2990632

You have chosen wisely.
You will continue
to do so.
Doubt whom you will,
but never yourself.

- Tom and Tipper

When conversing with your
invisible guides,
silently,
you will be heard.
You are
never alone.

- Perseus

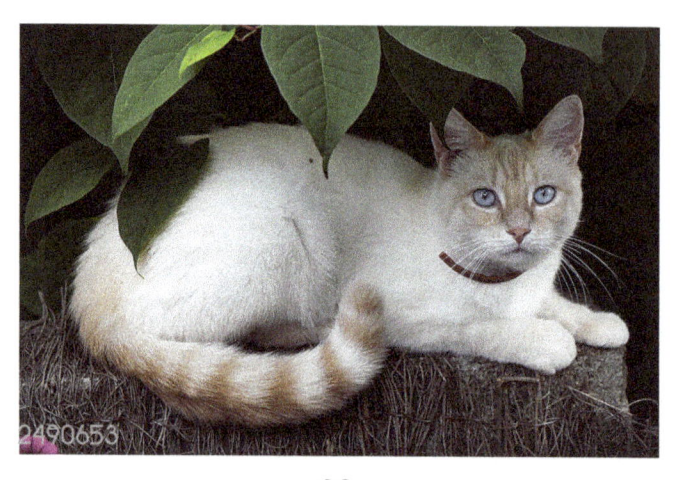

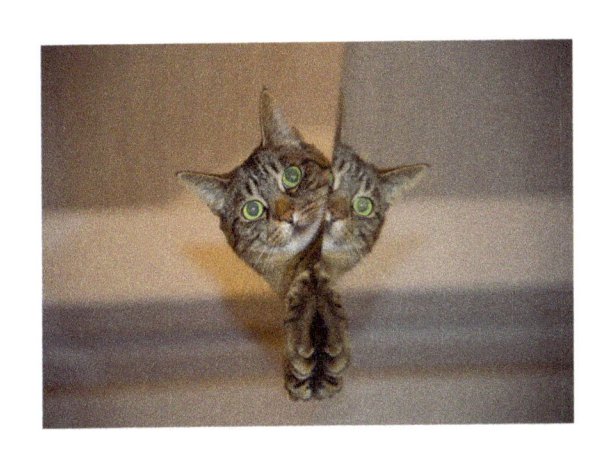

Be loud about your thankfulness, over and over. Praise is foreign to some. They may not realize how much they mean to you, even if you show them.
Repeat. Repeat.

- Tranquil

Forgive others as
soon as possible.
What you do not forgive
you carry. And hide.

- Androcles

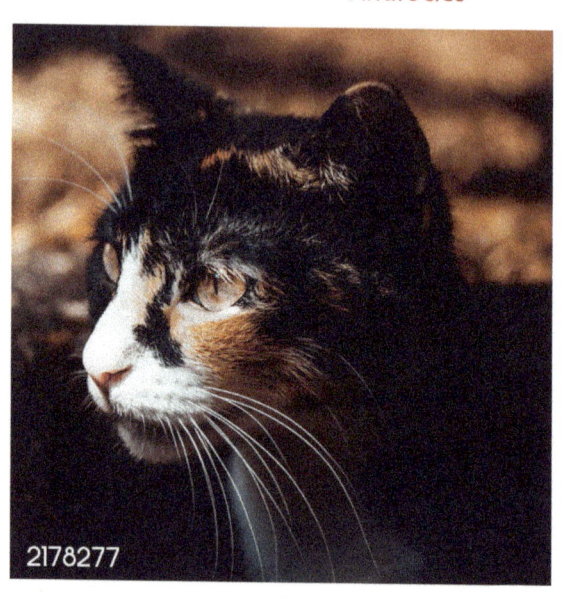

2178277

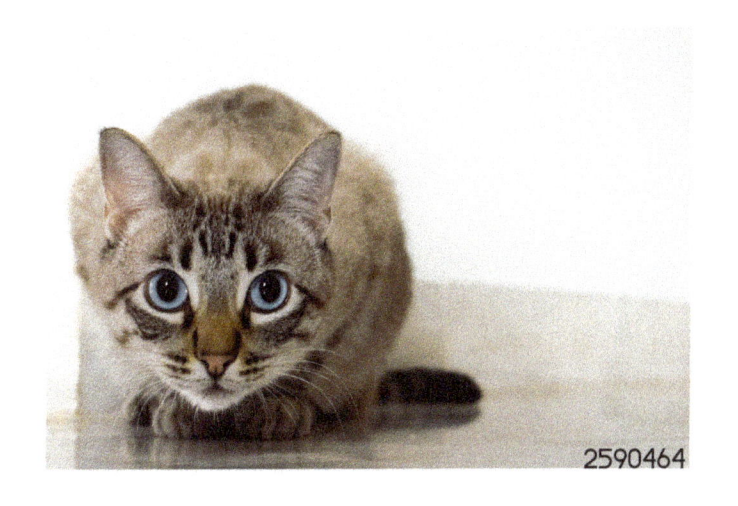

2590464

Center yourself
before leaping.
Centering is most
of the fun.

- Sapphire

While you are sleeping,
you are reviving.
Allow yourself to sleep
just like you did when you
were a kitten.
This is a real cat nap.

- Boris

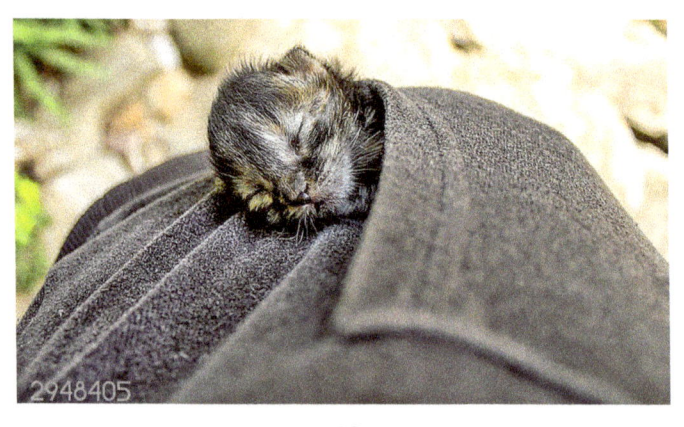

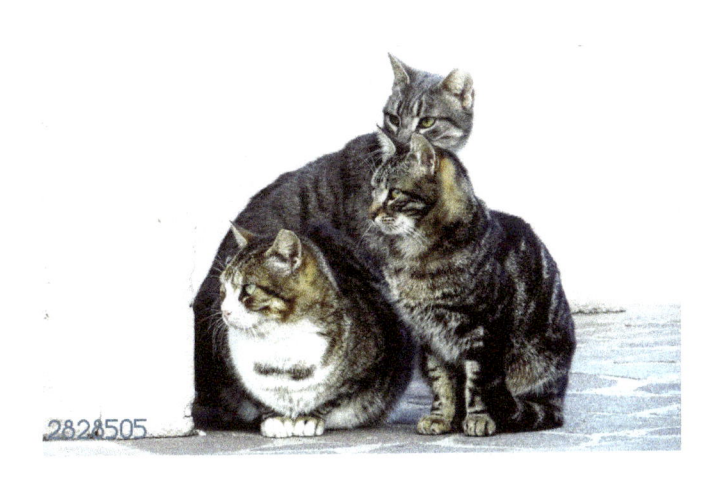

2828505

Reach out and play with others.
See what can happen.
Together, it's much more
enjoyable.
Learning to celebrate
anything
is a good start.

- Draper Crew

All of us do things
stupidly at first.
It's amusing.
Intelligence,
in many forms,
is so boring.

- Chacha

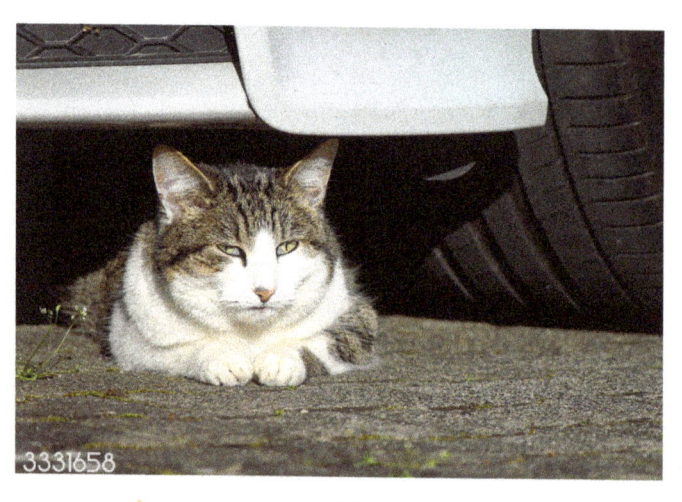

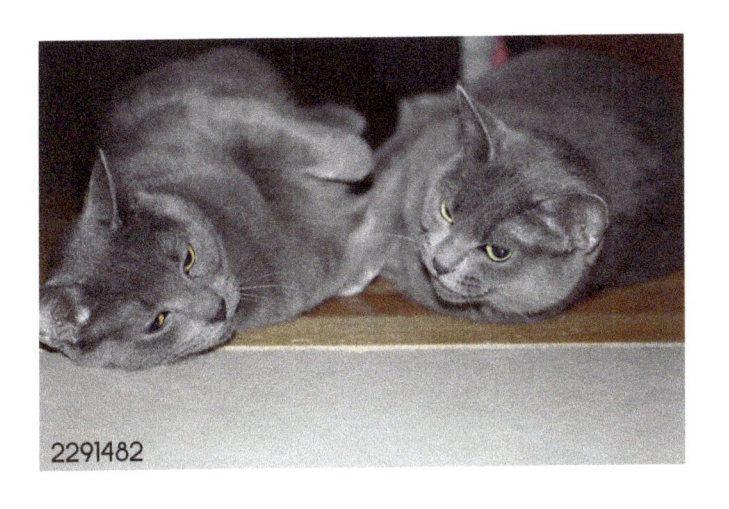

2291482

Bow to no one,
but honor those
deserving
with quiet dignity.

- Eve and Badria

Scan your body daily to
see what works.
Things change.
You are healing.
That's what a CAT scan
is all about.

-Tumm

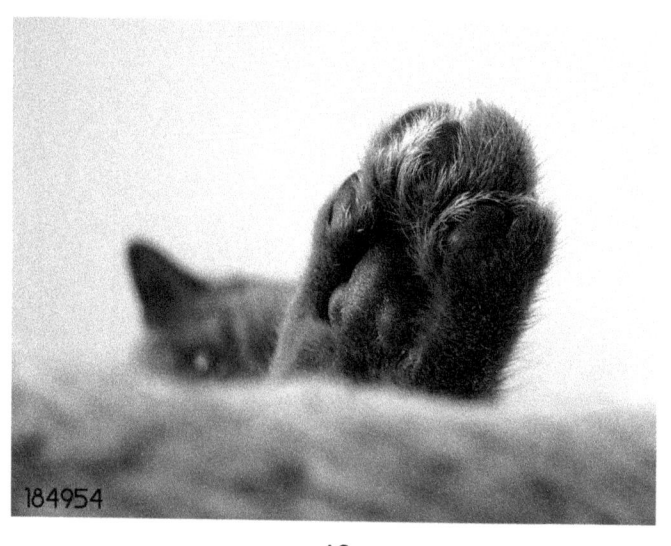

184954

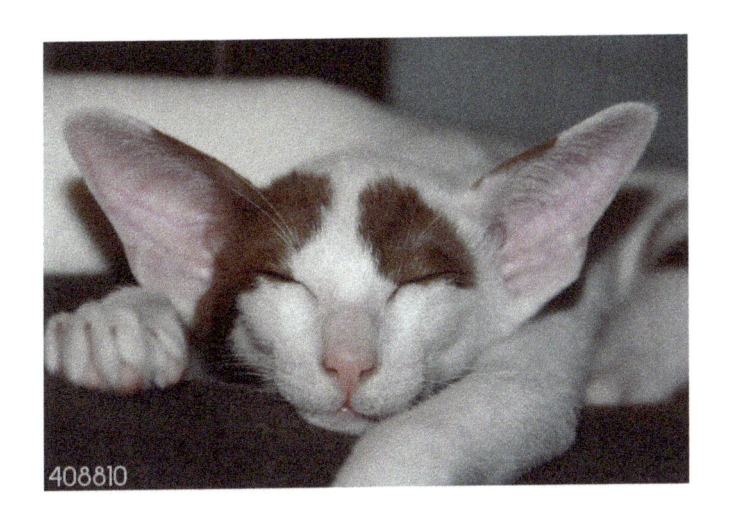

Don't be fooled by
any drug,
even if it's catnip
and everyone else
thinks it's
soooooo cool.

-Ayah

Do nothing against
your nature to
please another
but do things
you secretly enjoy
every day.

- Beauty

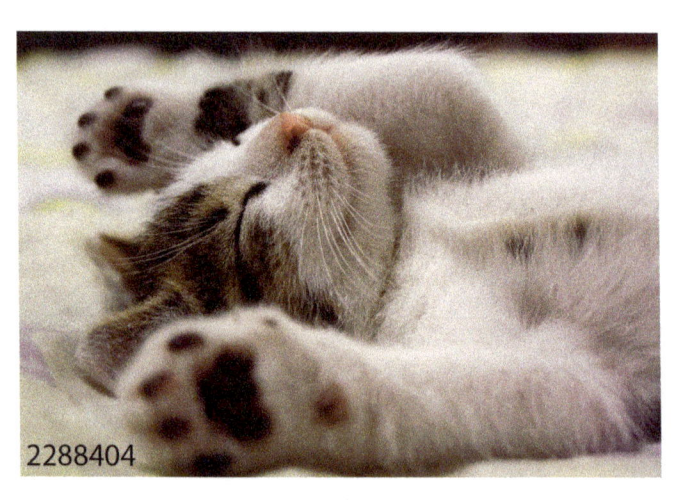

2288404

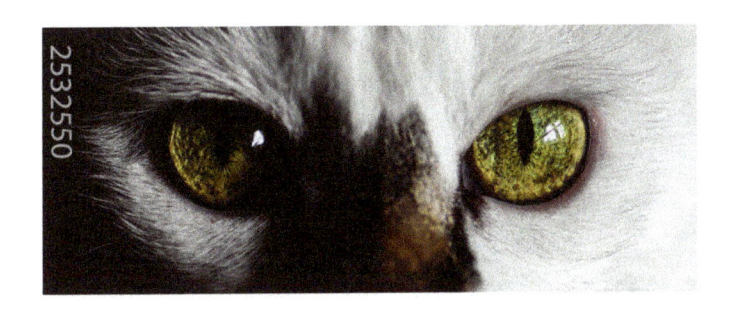

Apologize to no one.
Well, unless there
was a broken bone
involved.
Forgive yourself
with every breath.

-Yesh

Go slow most of the time and
relax into your curiosities.
Good things have a surprising
habit of appearing
all on their own,
sometimes after we just
open a door.

- Ophelia

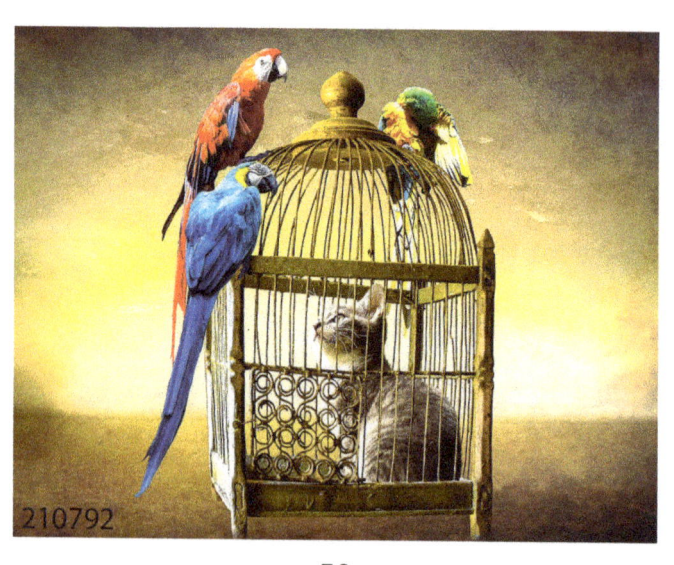

210792

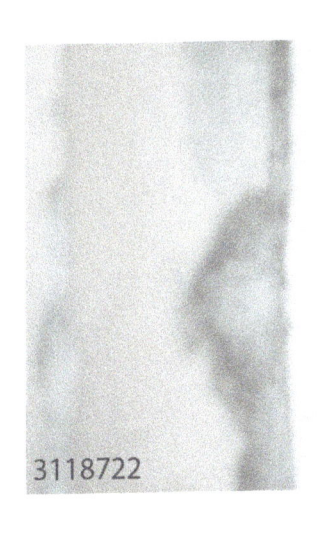

3118722

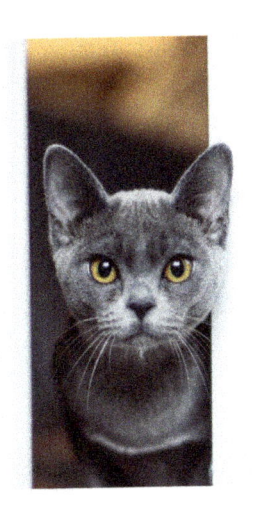

Set boundries and be
clear about them
especially with others.
Very clear.
You can thank
yourself later.

- Sienna

Listen to your favorite music and synch into your own rhythm. Sometimes you will see colors, but only with your eyes closed.

- Luna

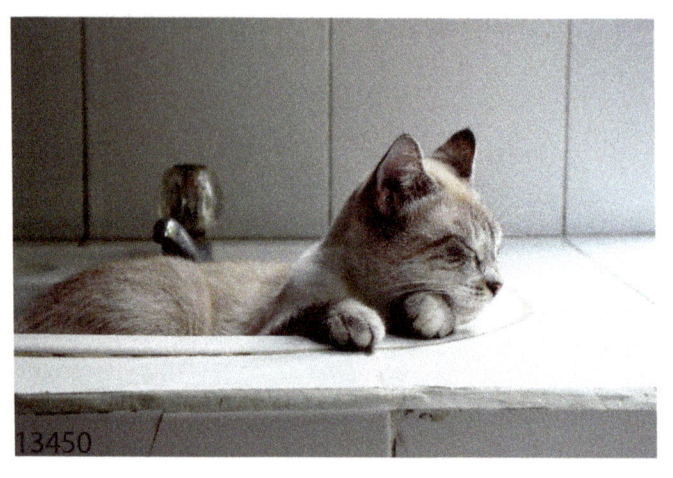

13450

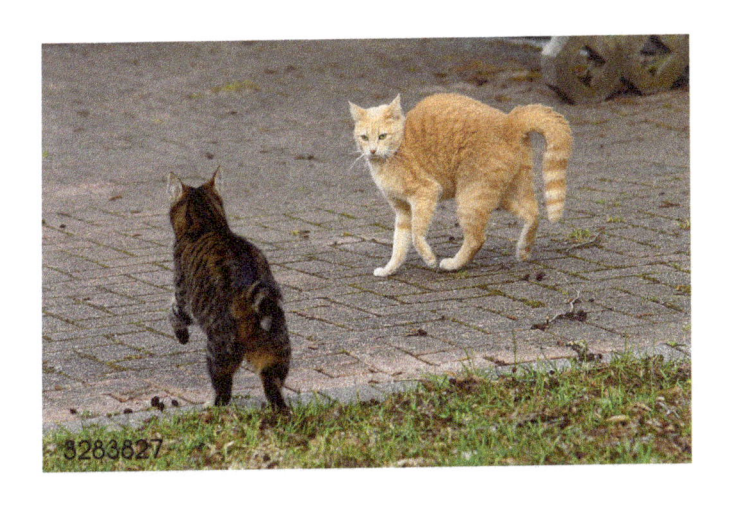

There's a reason for an
arched back and
a good hiss.
Scare away
enemies rather than fight.
Of course.

- Turk and Trudy

Trust yourself.
Trust your decisions.
You are still here because
you did that in the past.

– Bosco

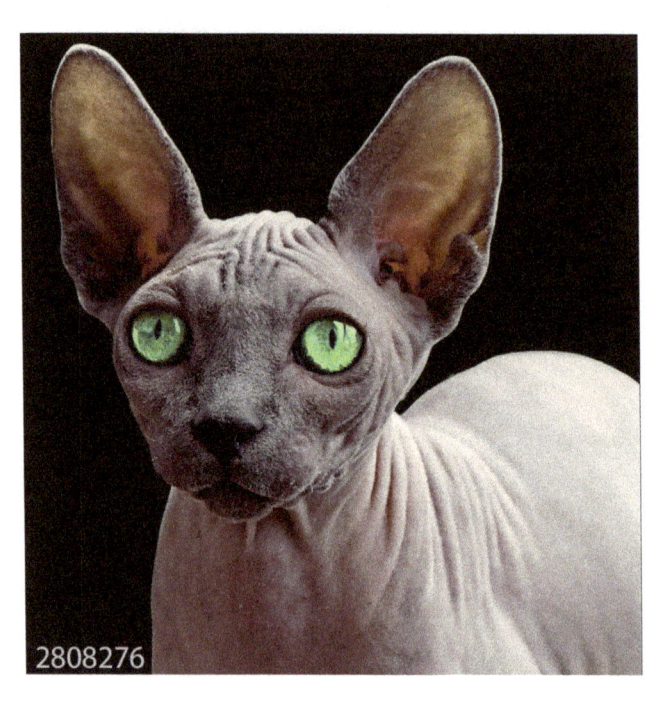

2808276

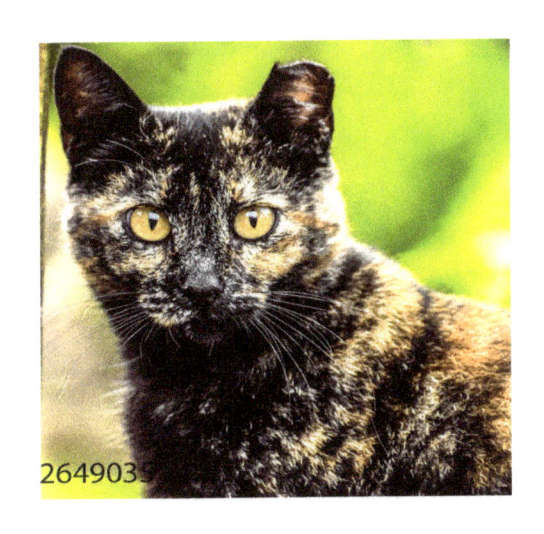

264903

You possess great knowledge and even greater power. In order to see it in others, you must see it first in yourself.

-Tele

Large challenges are made
of small ones.
Face the small ones
as if they were games.
Then stare down
the large ones.

- Francine

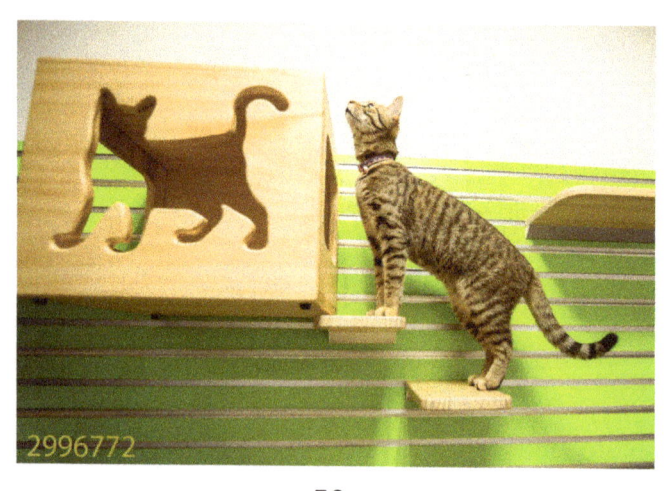

2996772

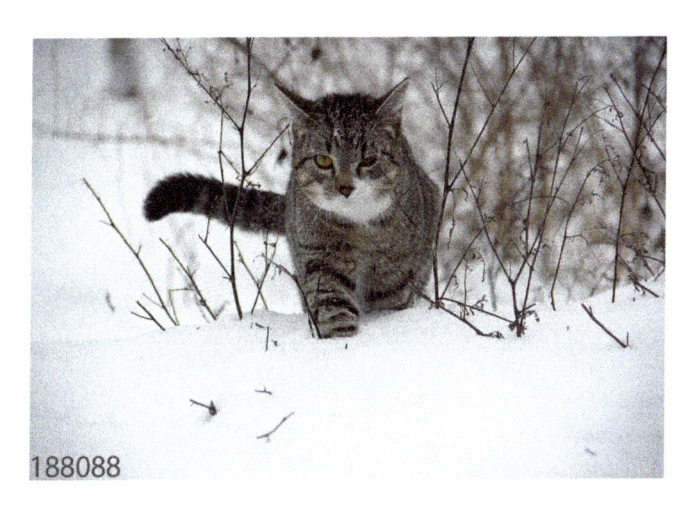

188088

Do not apologize for living your way. Even if some question your sanity. They are not housed inside your body and have not your experience nor your imagination.

- Lurch

Sleep where you want,
how you want
and with whomever
you want.

- Sweetie and Goldie

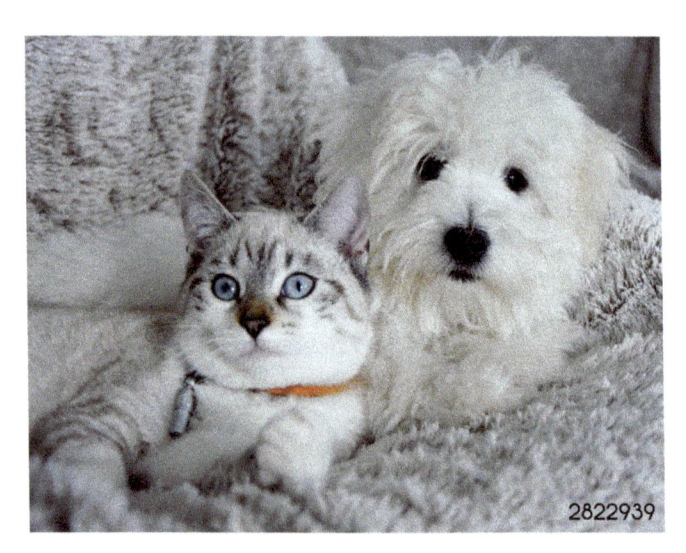

2822939

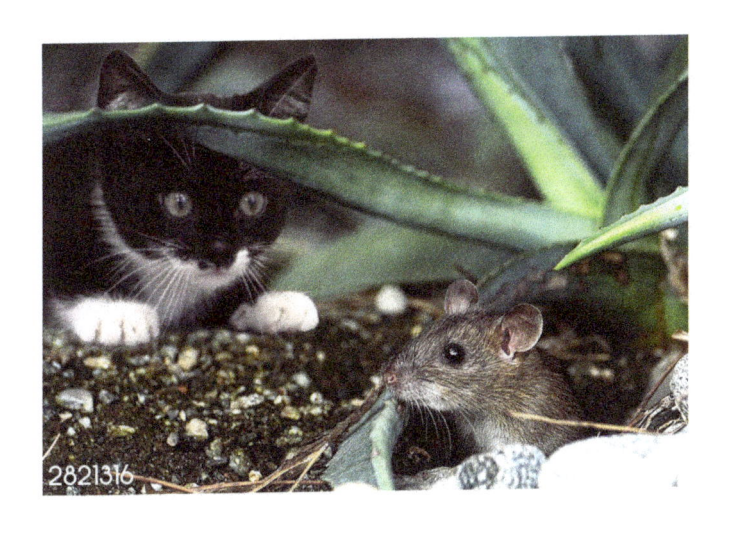

Nap, stretch, eat, leap,
drink, nap, stalk, listen.
Repeat.

- Kurious

Just as every blade of grass and
grain of sand is in the right place,
so is every single hair on your
beautiful body. You are perfect.
Laugh or weep when
you realize this,
but accept it as the truth.

- Gizmo

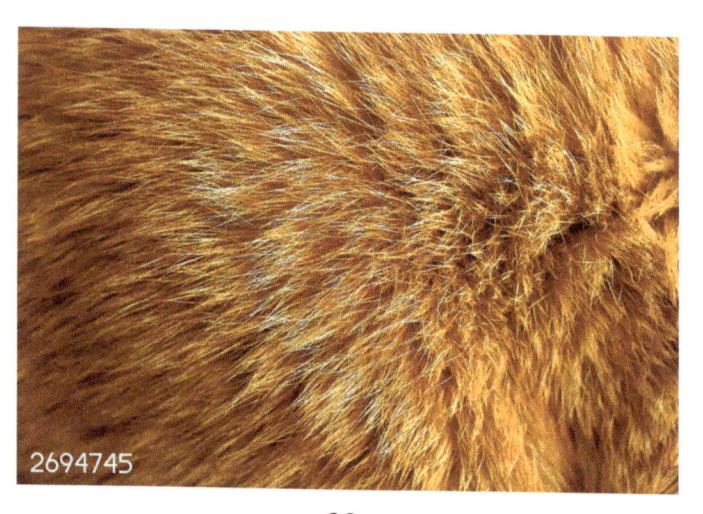

2694745

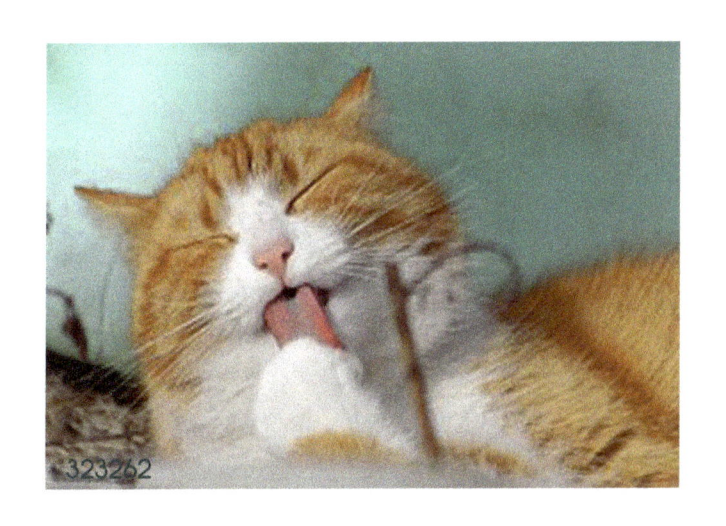

Stay groomed,
by yourself or with help.
Cough up the bad stuff.
This will happen
automatically.

- Lucinda

Place your feet carefully
with each and every step.
The slower you go
the faster you
will get there.

- Jazzy

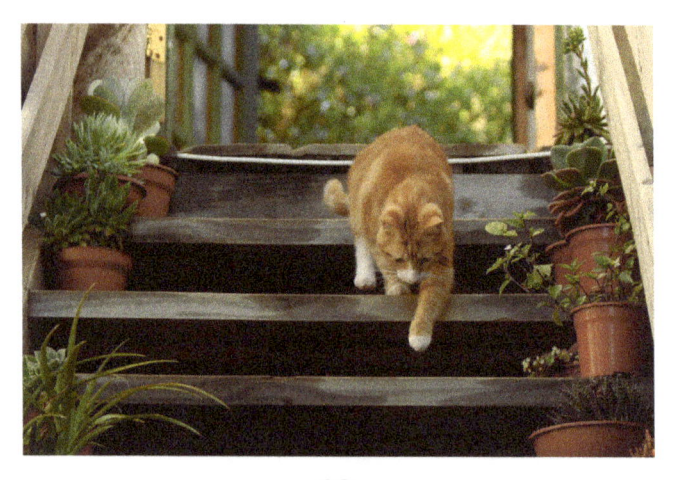

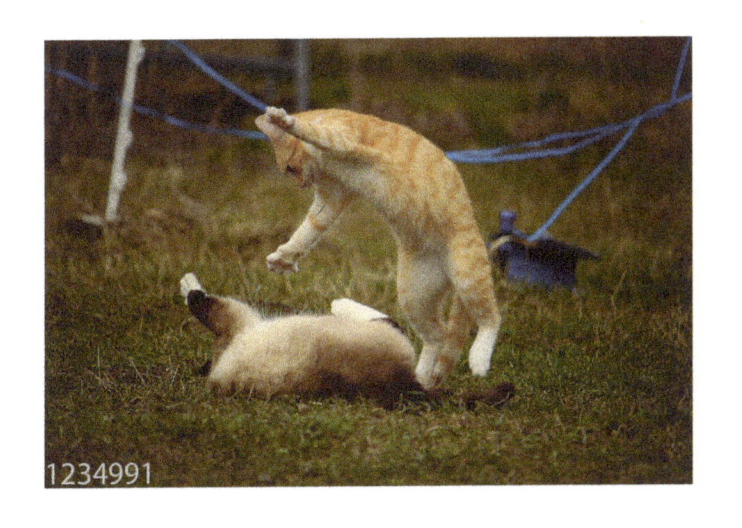

When you go fast,
forget about your feet
completely.

- Tucker and Turbo

If your family is mean,
intrusive or toxic, no need to fight.
Find your own tribe.
This may be difficult,
but keep searching.
Someone is looking for you too,
probably high up in a tree.

- Eyelet

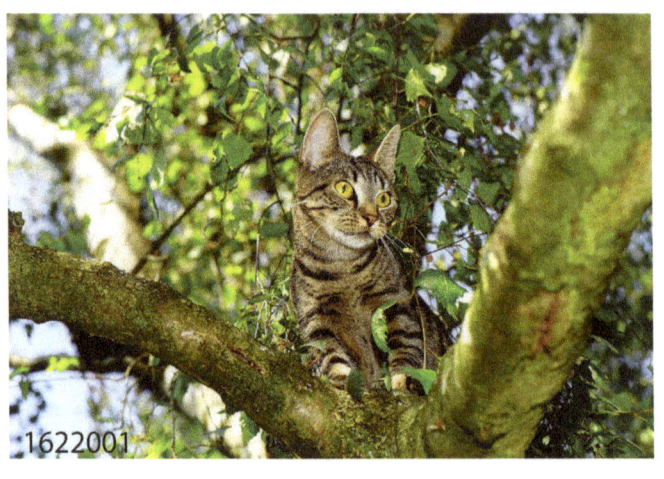

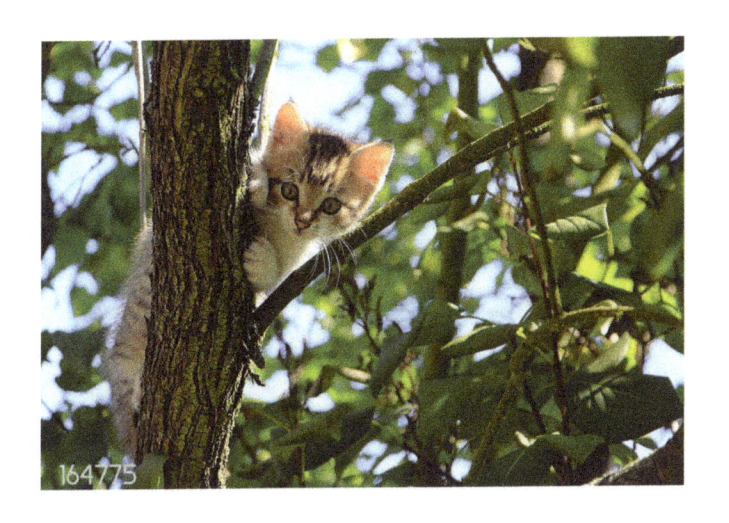

It takes a while to see
with perspective.
Being high up in a tree
is good for that.

- Cupid

While focusing, you may
become distracted.
Let the distraction pass.
Then return to this singular moment.
Otherwise you might
find yourself high
up in a tree forever.

- Raven

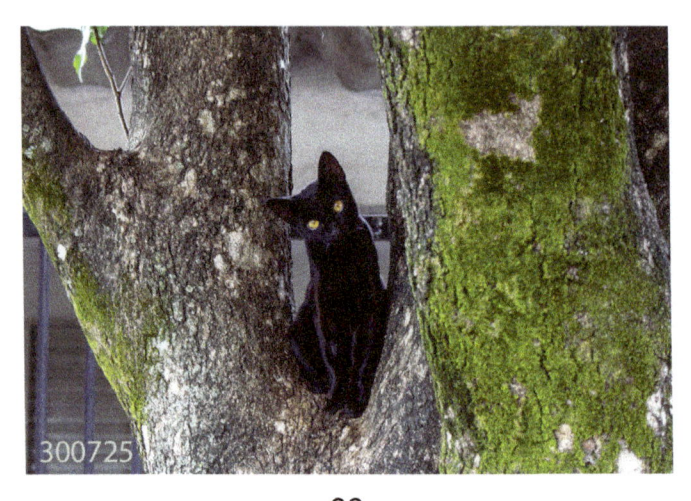

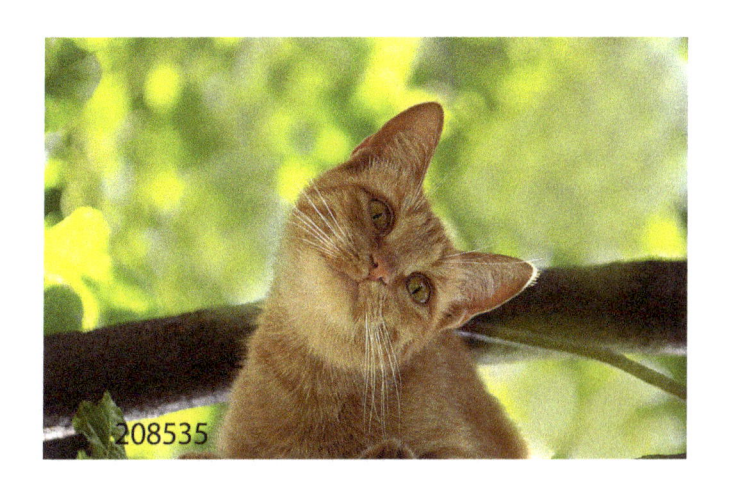

208535

When conundrums appear,
consult with your invisible guides.
What they say
might not make sense at first.
Slow down and take it in,
knowing you will get it.
Eventually.

- Spencer

Nervousness serves
no one.
Good and bad, in general,
do not exist.
They are temporary labels.

- Agent

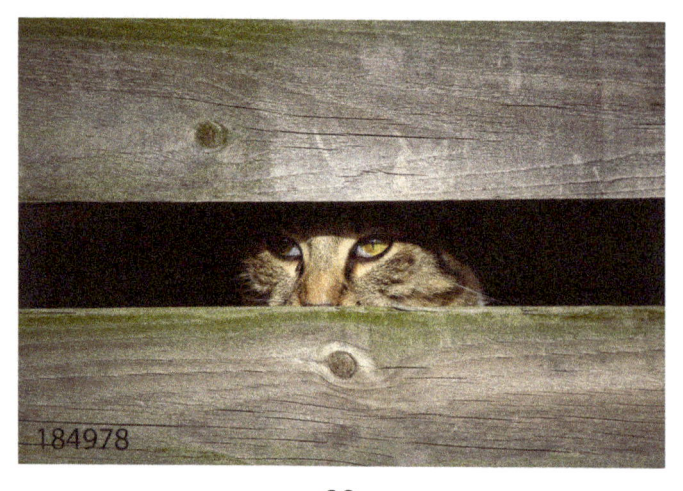

184978

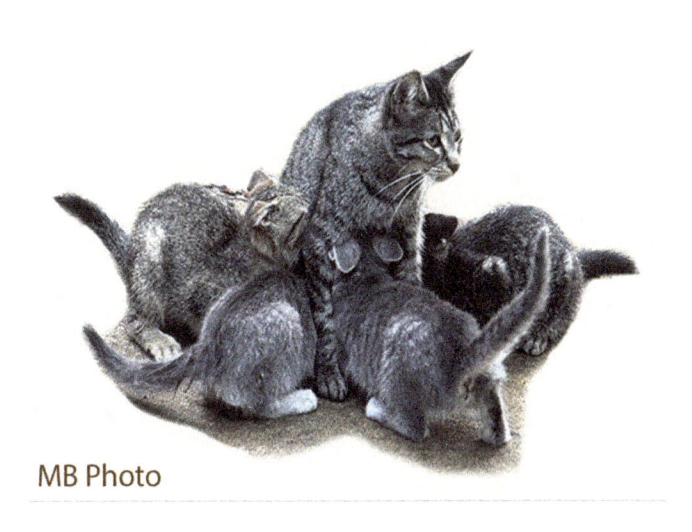

MB Photo

Do what is necessary to revive. No chasing mice, no jumping on the top of doors, no nursing kits just because they want to.

-The Kelsey Family

Stay close to the things
you love.
Lean into them.
This is the
truest of joys.

- Spike and Ursula

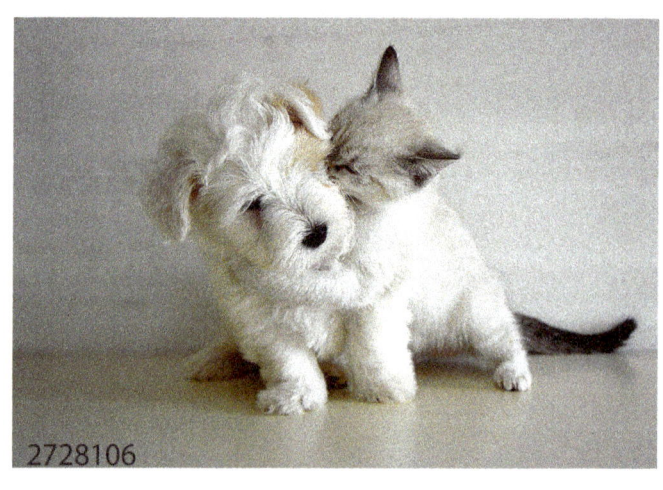

2728106

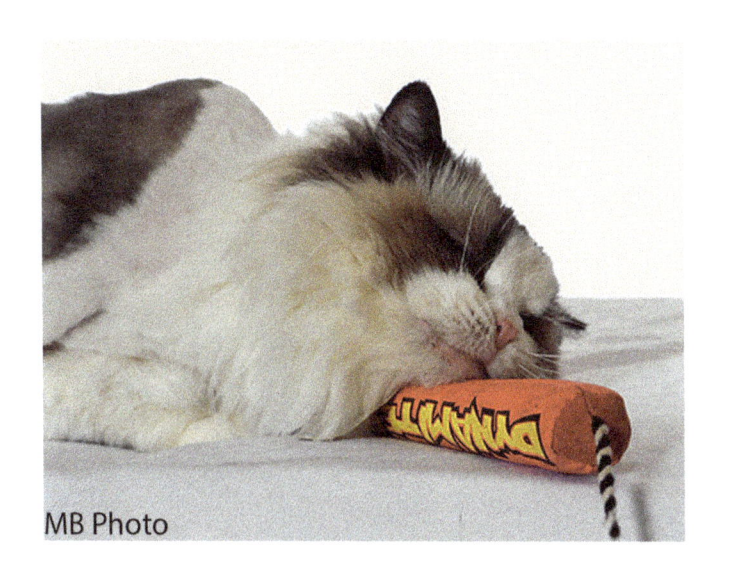

MB Photo

Leap vertically only
when you deem it
necessary.
It won't be that often.

- Venus

Speak in your own
unique voice.
Assume, occasionally,
that you will be heard.

- Calico

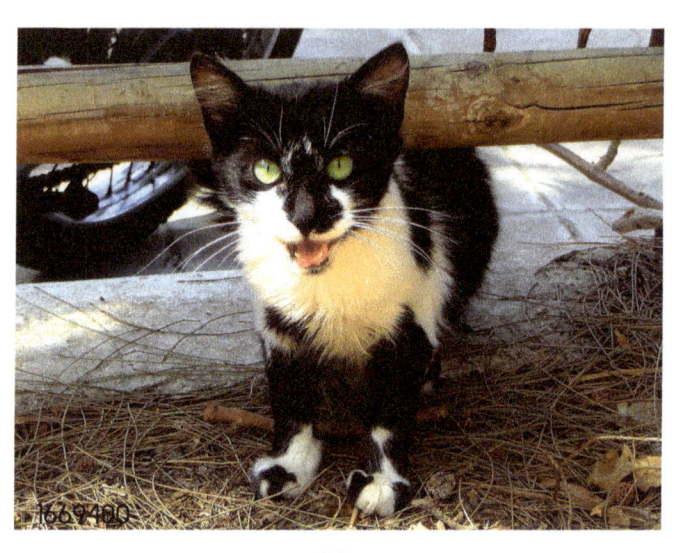

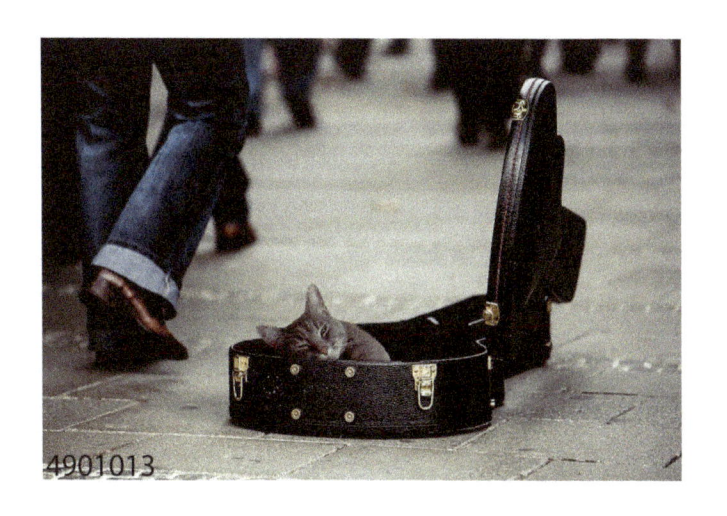

4901013

Plain, brown, square
boxes are not the only
cool thing in the world.
Open yourself and
find out what is open
and ready for you.

- Jules

Sometimes it may not
seem so, but truly all
choice is yours, almost all
the time.
That's enough.

-The Sunshine Crew

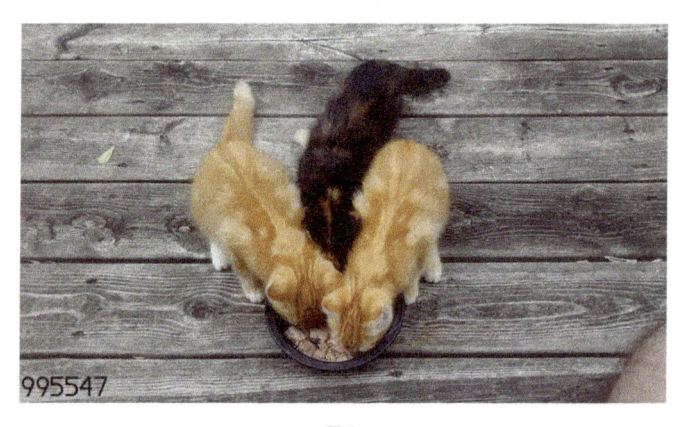

995547

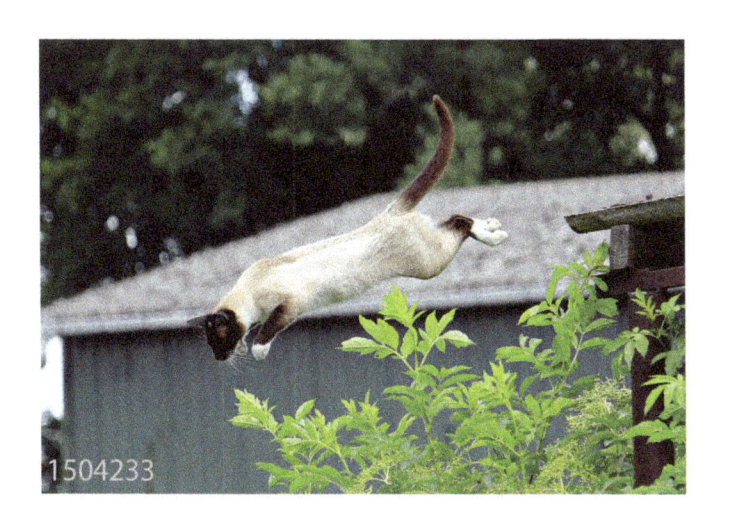

Sometimes it is
okay to go ahead
and leap.

- Dubhan

Timing is
Everything
and
Everything
is in
Perfect Timing.

- Dusty

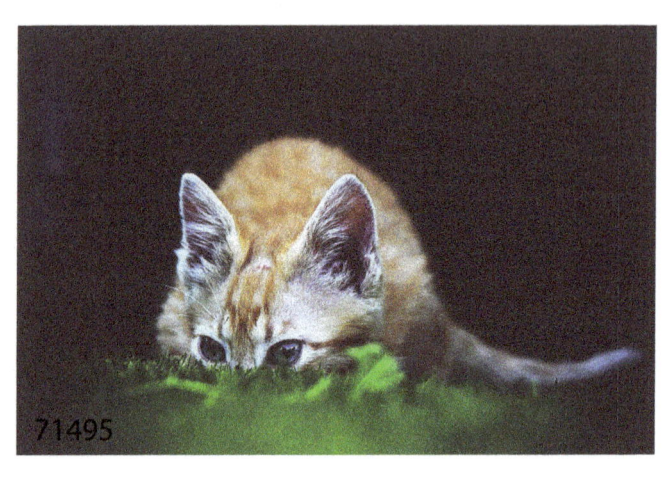

71495

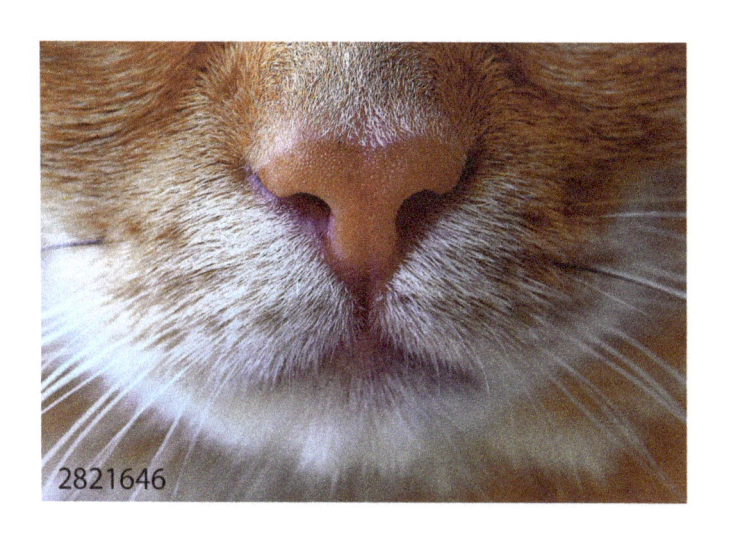

2821646

You are a part
of all the
beauty you see.

- Peachy

Hold on, but gently.
You've got this.

- Simon

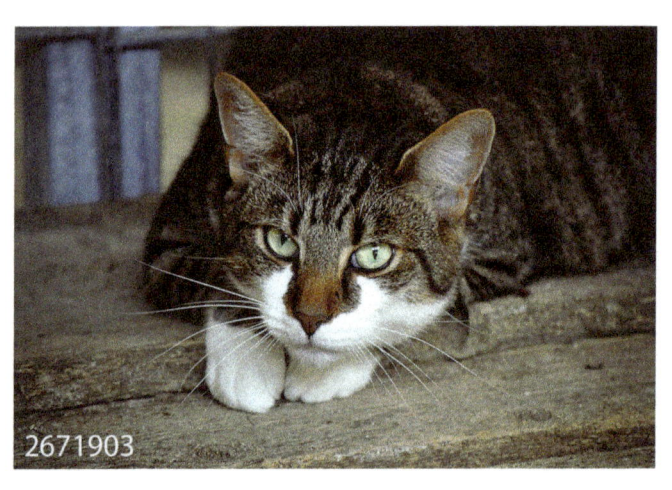

2671903

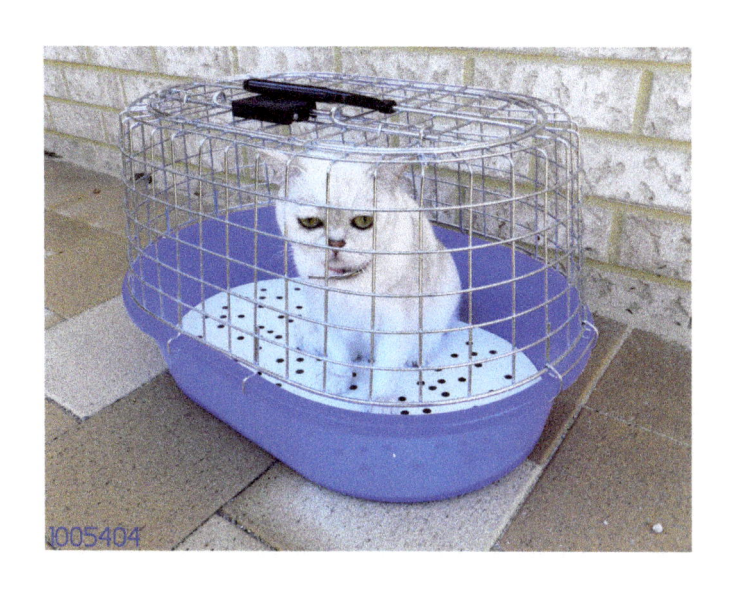

We are always in
the right place
at the right time
doing the right thing.

- Trixie

Float on the watercourse,
and always downstream,
there is nothing for you
upstream.

- Esther

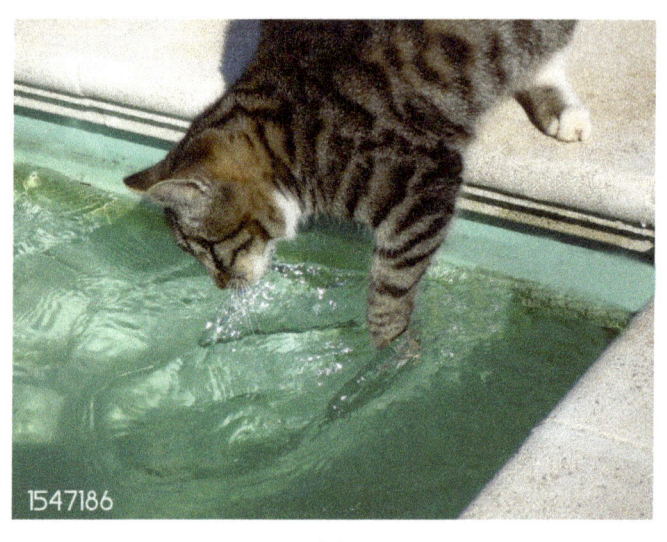

1547186

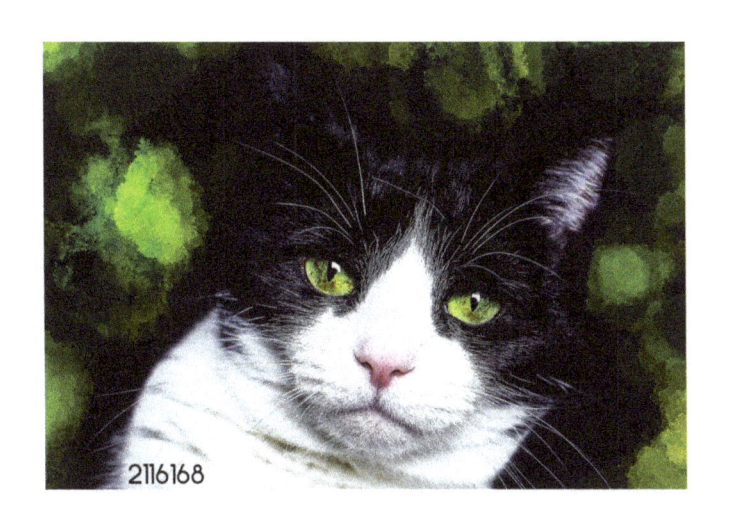

2116168

No hurry,
no worry necessary.

- Hasselworth

Forgetting works.
Remembering
is a gift.

- Andrew

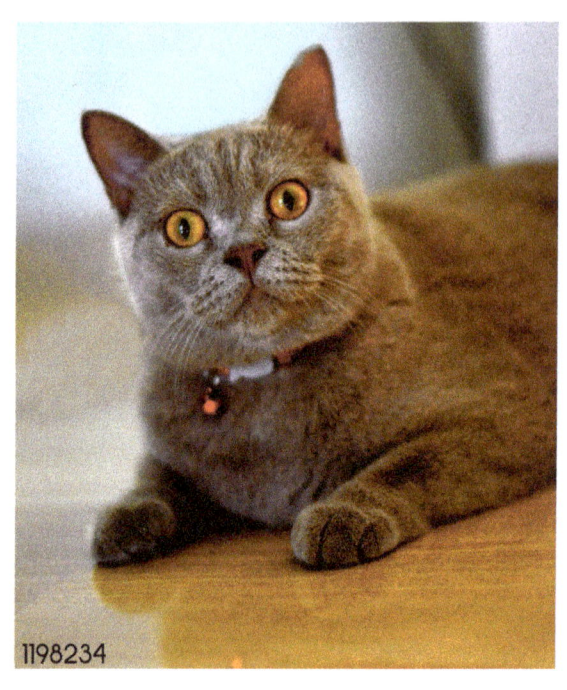

1198234

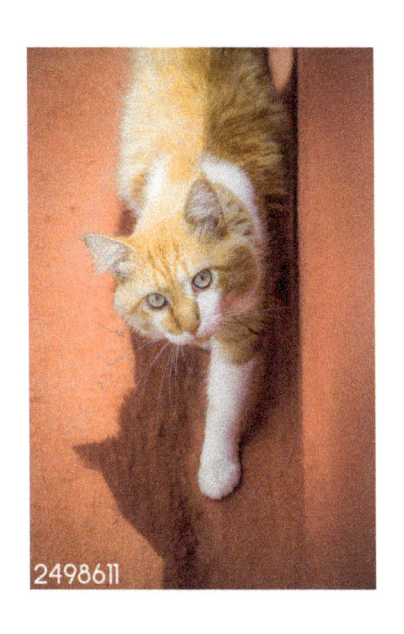

2498611

Send it away if there
is no benefit.
Or just walk in
another direction.

- Loretta

There's nothing wrong in giving up, for minutes, hours or even days. But if you are still here, after giving up, then there's more work and play to be done.

- Maxie

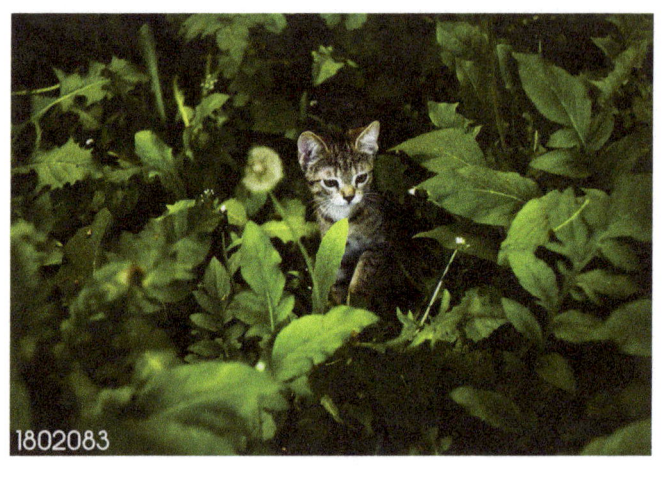

1802083

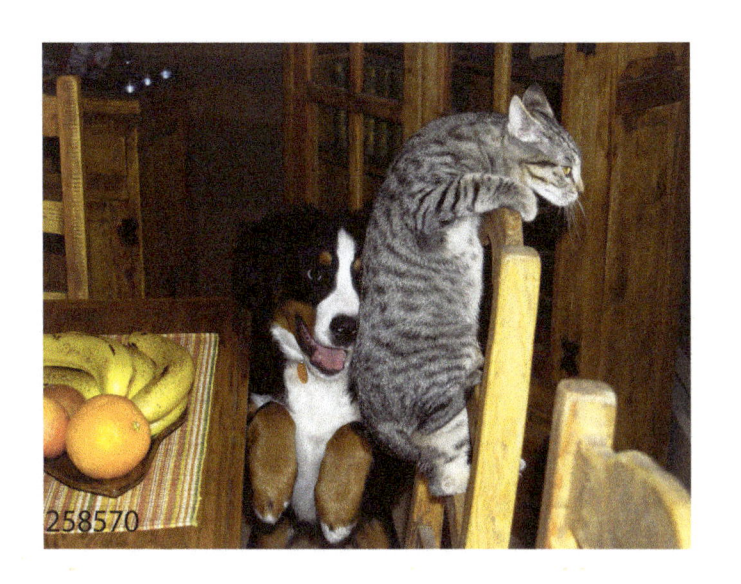

First comes chaos, then change, then calm. Celebrate the chaos because without it there is no creation, evolution or healing.

- Raleigh

Clear the path.
One can do much more
when there are
no obstacles.

- Charlie

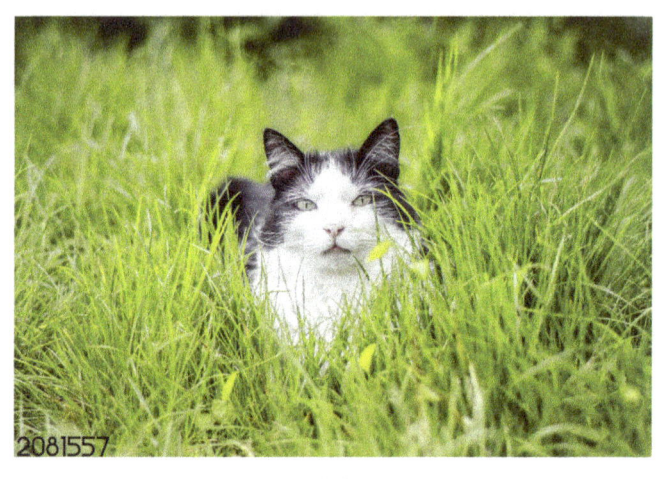

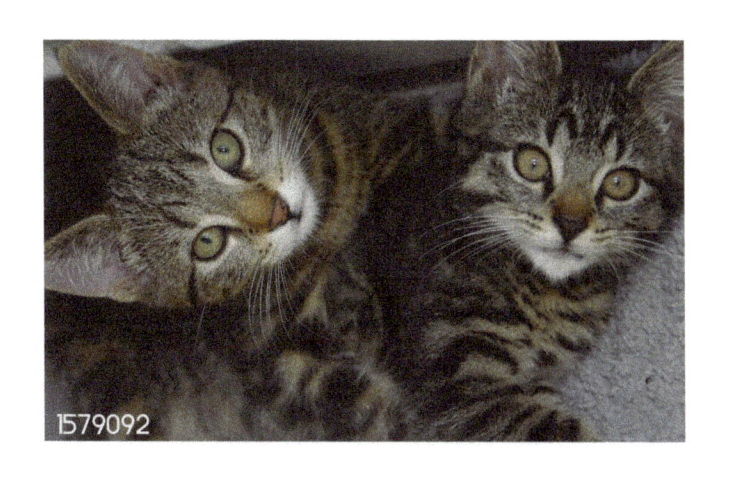

1579092

We can do more
together than we
can ever do alone.

- Gina and Gentry

Change nothing about you,
unless you want to.
Accept everything about
them just as they are.
And watch the
progress continue.

- Milo and Murphy

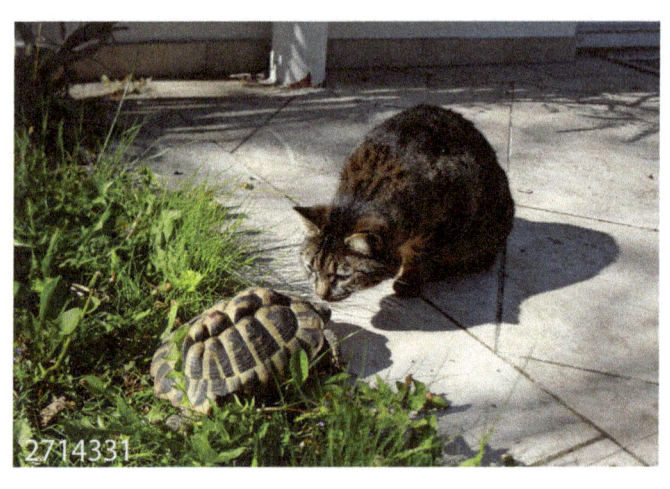

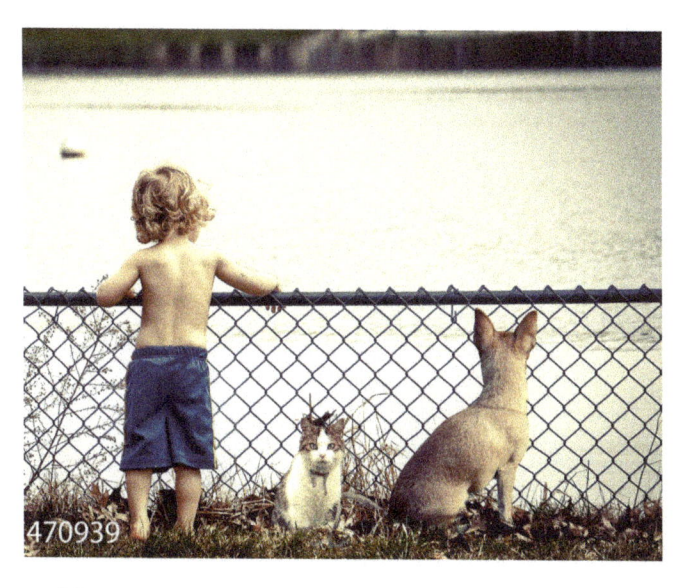

Mice, dogs, humans, fish
are all put here to make
us laugh on the inside,
while we are healing
on the outside.
Aren't we lucky?

- Kobe

When you no longer
think you can go on
find another in a
deeper hole to console.

- Samson and Delilah

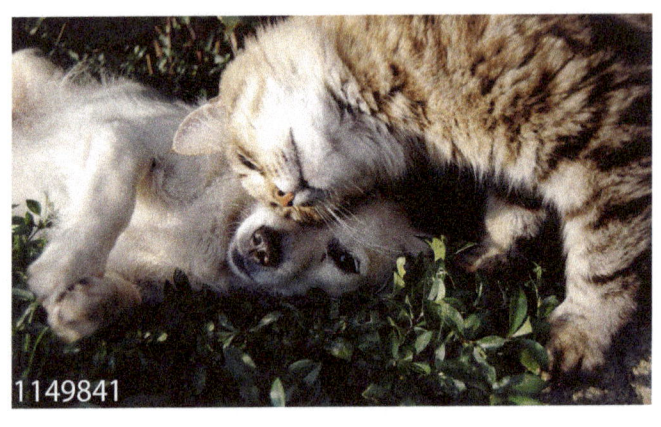

1149841

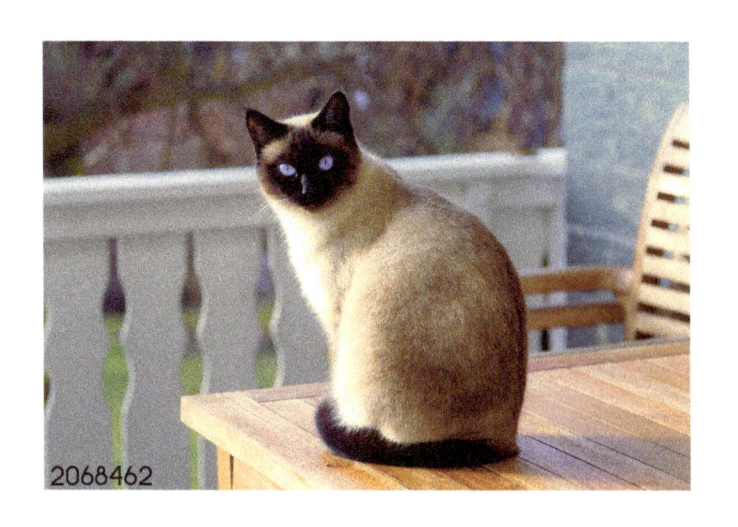

Stay focused on
what works.
Give nary a second
to what doesn't.

- Maggie

Extra anger and fear
have no business here.
Disperse and release
ASAP.

- Pawse

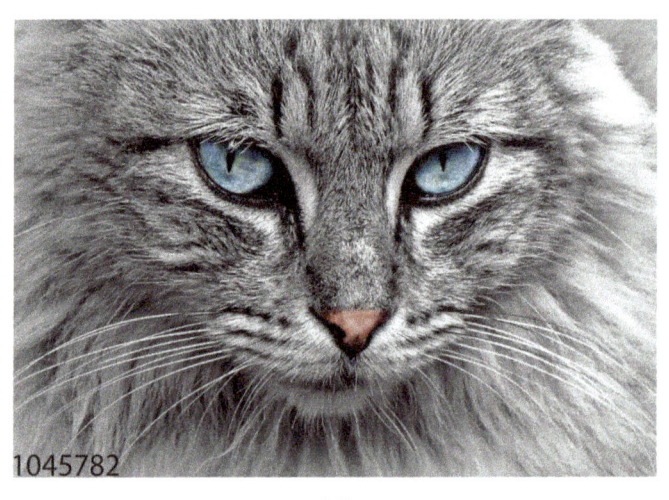

1045782

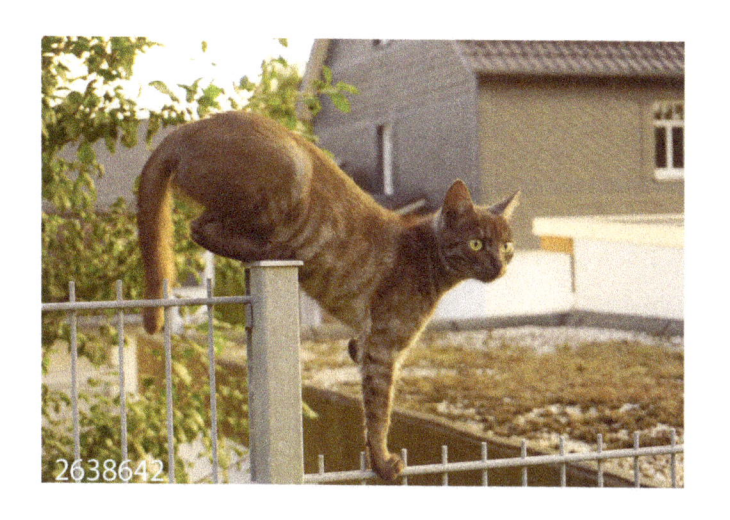

Balance has always
been the point.

- Buster

Pain reminds us we
are still alive.
Invite it to stay and
disperse all the other
energy out to infinity.*

- Squeaker

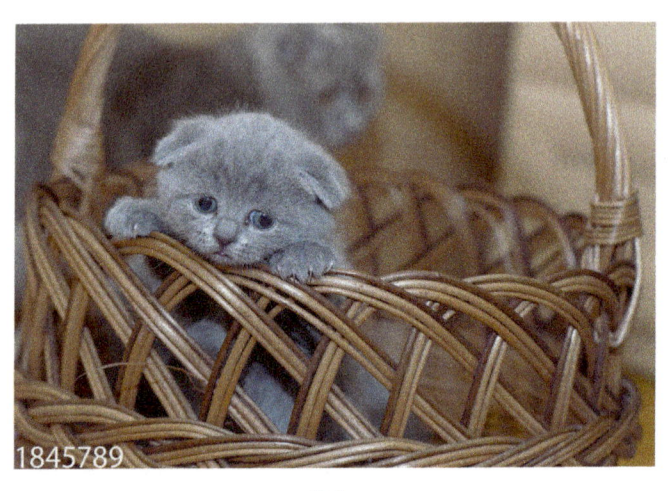

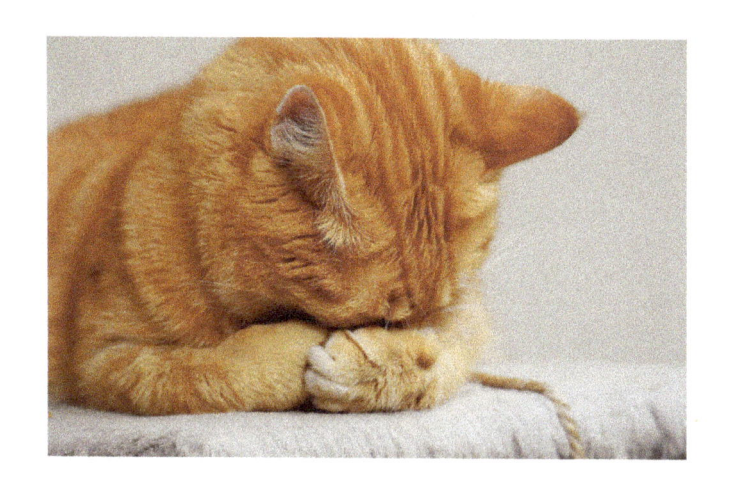

Read your own signs
since truly,
no one else can.

- Muffin

Charo kisses herself.
You may call it grooming,
but we call it self love.
Feel free to try it daily.*

- Freddie

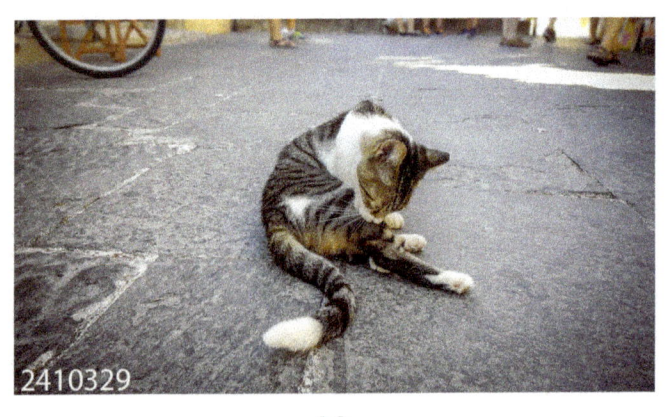

2410329

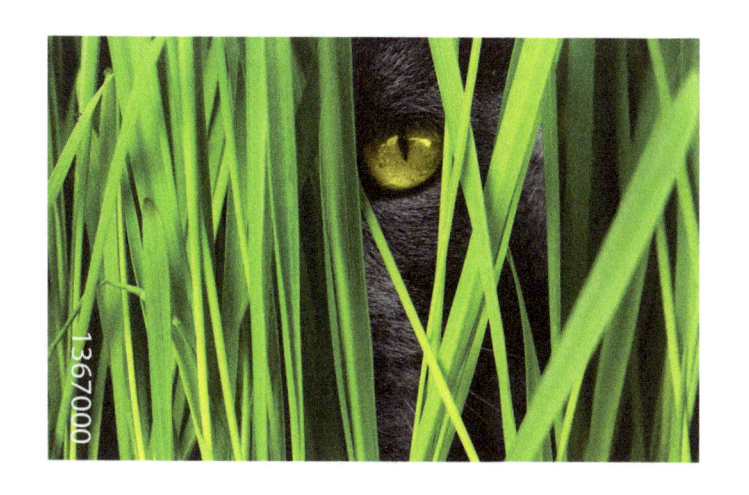

Kyle Cease talks to ghosts.
So do we. In both cases,
it's frustrating.
Better to stay on this
plane, even though
it's boring sometimes.*

- Fannie

Run around crazylike.
No one really cares.

- Kate and Kissy

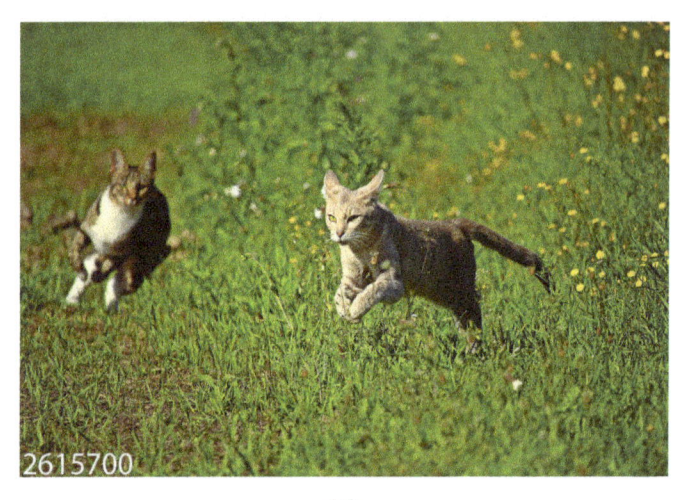

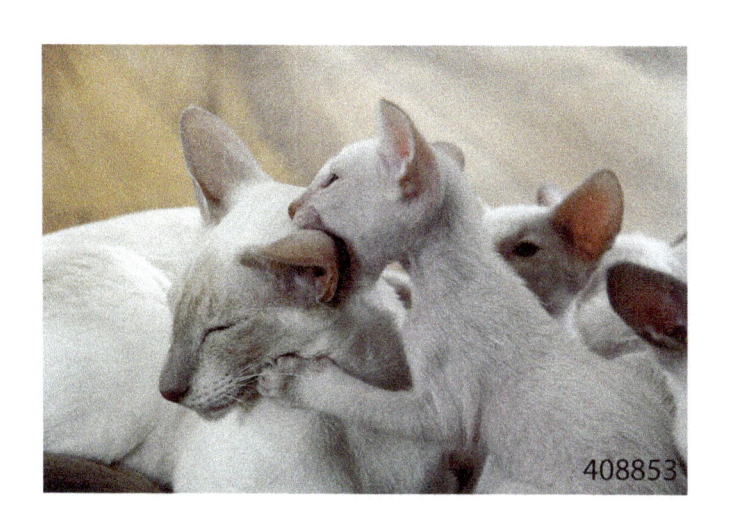

Do whatever it takes to
get their attention when
you need help or advice.
Gnaw on their ear.
Just don't bite down.

- The Casper Family

About the Author

Chris Collins wrote another book back in 2000 called Lemon Meringue Life which explained how to caregive for a high crisis individual. This was because she was caring for her seventeen year old severly brain injured son from an auto accident. After 14 years of caring for him, she became gravely ill and was told that unless she did immunosuppressive therapy (chemo) for her Aplastic Anemia, she would not live six months. Instead she went the route of Chinese medicine and after three months of bedrest and herbs began to feel better. That was over eight years ago.

About the Author (Cond't)

These days she credits meditation, a highly nutritious paleo diet and eliminating gluten, sugar and store bought milk products, adding in LDN, and trust that the Universe has her back for her consistently normal blood numbers in the past year. She wrote another book in 2015 called Beyond Terminal telling the story of how all that came about. She has done enormous research on how people with the 4th stage cancer, MS, ALS, blood disorders, and other diseases just keep living. Many of those people are listed on her website www.revivior.net.

About the Author (Cont'd)

and can be found in Kelly Turner MD's website "Radical Remission". In addition, there are people on her website who have survived car accidents, phenomenal surgeries, stroke and other amazing situations that one, at first, cannot even believe. In all cases she sees helpers of all types. She feels one's beliefs set the stage for healing and provide at least 50% of the solution. Her next book, Revivors! will come out in 2021 and will document those people who continue to show us how to heal, no matter what.

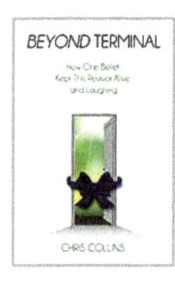

Beyond Terminal: How One Belief Kept This Revivor Alive and Laughing! Each year millions of people find themselves confronted with a word that is as frightening as it is hopeless. TERMINAL. When Chris Collins heard it for the first time, her world came crashing down around her. This book is founded on practical advice and brutally honest anecdotes, "Beyond Terminal" is a beam of light for those facing their darkest hour...

Lemon Meringue Life

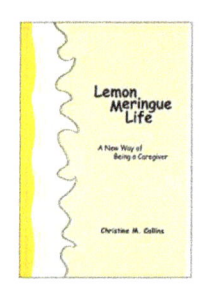

This book gives step by step instructions on planning for long term or short term caregiving, building Family Careteams and walking through crisis with hardly a scratch. Caregivers around the world have applauded Ms. Collins's work in putting down simple steps that can be used easily when facing family caregiving.

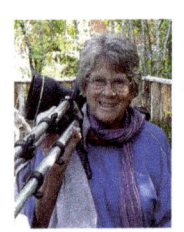

Marian Brickner
insect1@att.net

www.marianbricknerphotography.com

Marian Brickner, (b 1937) is an internationally acclaimed animal photographer, who began her distinguished career at the age of 55. Marian specializes in capturing specific individual moments in the lives of Bonobos (an endangered Great Ape), as well as insects, birds, dogs and cats through her stunning visual images. Her photos have graced the covers of books, appeared in National Geographic publications and been featured in calendars and billboards in France! She has authored or co-authored 38 books featuring her images, authored a documentary about Bonobos and participated in numerous gallery exhibits. Originally from New York Marian now lives in St. Louis, Missouri.

Marian Brickner Books on Amazon.com
Empathy series by Anne Paris

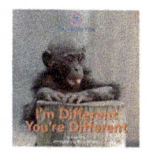 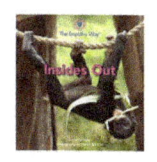 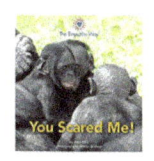 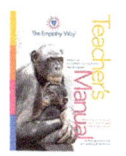

Bonobos Lucy and friends

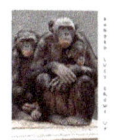 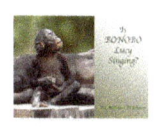 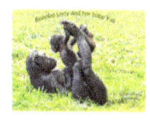 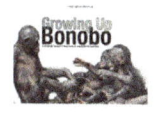

Books with Dogs ,Cats, Cartoons

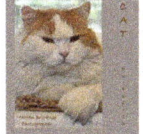 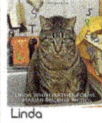 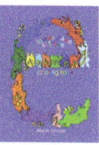 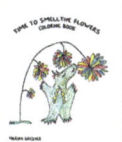 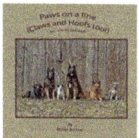

Birds and Bugs also

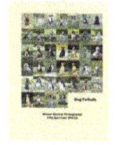 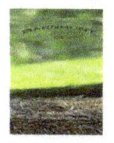 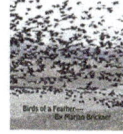 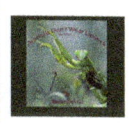 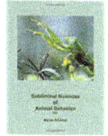

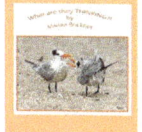 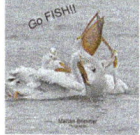 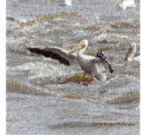 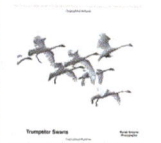

Good Websites

Marian Brickner
www.marianbricknerphotography.com

Amy Camie
www.healingharp.com

Kris Carr
www.kriscarr.com

Coleen Huber ND
www.natureworksbest.com

Lissa Rankin MD
www.lissarankin.com

Kelly Turner MD
www.radicalremission.com

Chris Wark
www.chrisbeatcancer.com

Website notes (Cont'd):

There are many hospitals, doctors and hospice centers to help you in your city if you want to go that route. In fact, too many to note here. But you will be able to find them easily. Looking for other options is something completely different and may take quite a bit more commitment as you walk your path. Whatever you feel is right for you, is correct. Use the coaches, docs, nurses and options that are available. Once you start on your journey back to health, you will find that the doors, just those made for you, will open. Trust yourself. Move forward. Keep going.

Final Accoutrements *

Kyle Cease is mentioned in the book because he talks to ghosts.
He has much to teach us and is an award-winning comedian and transformational coach. I send blessings to him every day.

Charo has long been a favorite of mine because she kisses herself all the time. I get that. I think we need more of that. Thank you Charo. Did you know she is an international flamenco guitarist? Oh, she is talented!

Final Accoutrements (Cont'd)

On page 94 we talk about inviting the pain to stay and sending the rest of the energy out in all directions to infinity. If you want to know how to do this, get the book, Open Focus by Les Fehmi. It has helped me through some pretty impressive dental work among other things. By the way, all of these thoughts are mine or have been given to me from who knows where, but I do believe in them and I think the cats would agree. Nothing is in concrete. Just employ the ideas to use or pitch, your choice.

Final Accoutrements (Cont'd)

May you be blessed and know how much you are loved.

Fun Stats on Cats!

1) A group of us is called a clowder. Could be worse.
A group of crows is called a MURDER!

2) A cat who stays is not a cat who sprays. We have to remember that.

3) A "scaredy cat" is more a case of excellent night vision, hearing and an acute sense of smell rather than being afraid. So there.

Fun Stats on Cats! (Cont'd)

4) We never listen, never knock, but always come home. Hopefully bearing lots of mice and birds for your viewing pleasure.

5) Our tongue has backward facing spines, the better to groom ourselves with my dear. Or constantly kiss ourselves. We love us.

Fun Stats on Cats! (Cont'd)

6) We cannot taste sweets so don't give us those kind of treats. Or we will bite your feets.

7) The majority of us like to sleep 13-14 hours a day, up to 20. Be quiet or not. We love you anyway because we love family.

Fun Stats on Cats! (Cont'd)

8) We like to play with our prey to wear them out. Just like what you do with those dang lights on the wall. Whew!

9) From when we were kittens we pretended to fight. We don't really fight unless it's important, just like when mating season is here. Just sayin'.

Fun Stats on Cats! (Cont'd)

10) We like to perch on high places and we cannot lie. The easier to pounce on others and pretend to fly.

11) We tried to teach humans patience and it was almost as hard as teaching dogs to wag their tails slowly and with intent. Miserable failures both.

Fun Stats on Cats! (Cont'd)

12) Most countries say we have nine ives, but in Italy, Germany, Greece and Brazil they say 7. In Turkish and Arabic countries, 6. We believe we are immortal, of course.

13) Litter-ally it stinks in here! Change the litter often or the glare will be real.

Your Notes

Your Notes

Your Notes

Your Notes

Your Notes

CPSIA information can be obtained
at www.ICGtesting.com
Printed in the USA
FSHW021740061118
53435FS